£12·95

RA

Sustaining Sa

Social Aspects of AIDS

Series Editor: Peter Aggleton
Goldsmiths' College, University of London

Contents

Contents

Series Editor's Preface

When research into the social aspects of HIV disease began over a decade ago, it was often argued that surveys of knowledge, attitudes and sexual behaviour were a prerequisite for the design of effective interventions. In retrospect we have learned that such claims were but partially true, since while such research held the potential to inform HIV and AIDS-related health promotion, only rarely did it do so effectively. Moreover, numerous interventions have been planned and effected using knowledge of a quite different kind — that gathered locally from smaller groups of people using more qualitative, open-ended and ethnographic techniques. Of course, the most effective kinds of health promotion are those which have their foundations in both of these kinds of research — the quantitative to identify overall trends, patterns and relationships within a given population; the qualitative to provide insight and understanding into the cultural processes which shape and constitute risk-related relationships and practices.

It is against this backcloth that we must position a book such as *Sustaining Safe Sex: Gay Communities Respond to AIDS*. For with remarkable foresight, the authors recognized the need to combine together different research techniques in the pursuit of knowledge to guide intervention planning. They saw too the productive way in which a non-individualistic social theory might inform an understanding of the ways in which behaviour change might be brought about and sustained.

While the book's focus is on the cultural processes at work within Australian gay communities before and after AIDS, the analysis offered has clear relevance to work in Europe, North America and elsewhere. As the authors argue, to conceptualize safer sex as a community rather than an individual practice is to rethink our approach to the determination of HIV-related risk. It is, moreover, to identify new intervention options where previously choices seemed limited. And it is to value positively the contribution gay men all over the world have made to our understanding of the epidemic and ways in which it might be contained.

Peter Aggleton

Preface

This book is based on the research of a team who worked together from 1985 to 1991 on the Social Aspects of the Prevention of AIDS (SAPA) project and its follow-up, the Sustaining Safe Sex (SSS) study. The researchers were psychologists and sociologists, statisticians, trained interviewers, members of the gay community, and workers at the AIDS Council of New South Wales, Australia. As our basic aim was to help educators and others working in organizations whose constituency comprised those most at risk of HIV, our first responsibility was to communicate with, and to inform, such organizations and institutions.

To this end we evolved — rather than planned — a program that tried to deal with these different demands. It had five main components:

1 a set of short data papers, which we called 'technical reports' (perhaps not a well chosen name), mostly designed for HIV/AIDS educators and sometimes written in response to a specific request, e.g., for information about condom use or as background material for a training workshop (ten in all);
2 a series of monographs reporting the main data analyses, with each reporting a large 'chunk' of the data; the monographs, from thirty-three to fifty-five pages long, were an attempt at a thorough documentation of the study for a mixed audience of AIDS educators and researchers (eight in all, listed in the appendix);
3 papers for academic journals, based on the monograph series but condensed and rewritten as appropriate for journal publication (six in all), plus one book chapter;
4 presentations and workshops to HIV/AIDS educators (over thirty workshops have been conducted in four states); it is not

enough just to publish — it matters to work through the issues with the users, to make sure the research is being interpreted correctly, to find out what aspects of our work are useful and what are not; and

5 a varied but continuous round of consultations on research, evaluation and policy; conference and seminar presentations; committee work; writing other papers informed by SAPA; media contact, teaching and so on.

The process of dissemination continues, and more recently a number of our team have taken part in World Health Organisation sponsored meetings, consultations and technical working groups and discussed the successes and failures of our attempts to involve those from affected communities in the planning of HIV and AIDS research. This book is part of the same process.

The research has had the support of a team of interviewers, secretaries, clerks and typists without whom we would not have been able to work. It has also had the support of non-government organizations such as the AIDS Council of New South Wales and the Australian Federation of AIDS Organizations, as well as State and Commonwealth Health Departments and AIDS Bureaux and Units. The Social Aspects of the Prevention of AIDS study was funded by the Commonwealth and State Departments of Health. Later research has been funded, in the main, by Australian government agencies, especially the Commonwealth AIDS Research Grants Committee; we have also received funds from the non-government sector and from Macquarie University.

We wish to acknowledge and thank all those with whom we have worked and those who have been our co-researchers, our respondents. Especially we would like to thank Pam Rodden and Vicki Sinnott; without their help this study would not have been possible. We also thank those who have given us intellectual support and encouragement when we did things a little differently from the accepted and the tried: Dennis Altman, John Ballard, Don Baxter and Lex Watson.

Since our coming together in 1985, the Australian research community has recognized our work. The research is now housed in the National Centre for HIV Social Research, one of three national HIV/AIDS research centres funded by the Australian government, and the only social research centre. At this third centre we have continued to work on the social aspects of the prevention of AIDS and have extended our research to those people living with HIV and AIDS. Most of our work has been directly concerned with sexual practice —

both homosexual and heterosexual — but we have also occasionally ventured to work with drug users.

We have learnt a great deal about HIV and AIDS, about education and prevention, and about the role of community in bringing about change. We have also learnt a great deal about sexuality, our own and that of others.

Susan Kippax, R.W. Connell, G.W. Dowsett and June Crawford

Chapter 1

Introduction

This book is about a research program concerned with the social aspects of the prevention of AIDS. We called it the Social Aspects of the Prevention of AIDS (SAPA) project. It details the development, the doing and the results of the research project, the process involved in each stage of the project, and the follow-up study, Sustaining Safe Sex (SSS).

At the outset of the research at the end of 1985, it had been clear for some years that the only way of stopping the HIV epidemic was by social action: by a combination of education programs, collective action by affected groups and well designed public services. This remains true today, some eight years later. In terms of conventional medicine there is no 'cure' for AIDS, and at the time this research began there was little by way of treatment. It would seem, then, that the most relevant kinds of research were, and are still, social scientific: research which focuses on the way of life in populations and groups where infection has spread, on the cultural context which shapes people's understandings of the disease and practice in response to it, and on enabling the adoption of effective preventive strategies.

The field of HIV/AIDS research was colonized from the start by medical discourse — a discourse of 'cause' and 'cure', of 'prevention' and 'treatment', of 'intervention', 'monitoring', 'risk groups' and 'risk categories' and so on. Had the question of *social action* been dominant from the start, we might have had a discourse derived from sociology, adult education and community activism instead. We might be talking 'needs analysis', 'curriculum', 'empowerment', 'networking', 'mobilization', 'reflexivity'. Perhaps we should make an effort now to change the vocabulary of AIDS-talk — at least to set this discourse alongside the medical one.

Willis (1983) has familiarized us with the idea of 'medical

dominance' in the social process of maintaining health. In the case of HIV/AIDS research we have a situation we would call 'medical hegemony'. Other perspectives and approaches exist; but they become marginalized by the dominant discourse, which is that of scientific medicine. Thus when the social sciences are called in, they tend to be set low-level questions (e.g., to count risky behaviours; to measure the impact of an information campaign). This is partly because these are the items wanted in a medically framed research/action agenda; and partly because the wider capacities of the social sciences are simply not known to medically trained researchers and administrators. One must also acknowledge, however, that the social sciences have not made a strong showing in this field even in their own terms. There are conceptual and technical problems. Four major weaknesses of this body of social research are immediately obvious.

First, there is frequent reliance on 'samples' which are essentially opportunistic; they sample nothing in particular and do not tell us anything about a definable *population* or *situation*. There seems often to be confusion between a *clinical series* and a *sample survey*; between epidemiological research and social analysis; between prospective studies of infection and community studies of a social group. A bizarre moment dramatized this point when in planning the SAPA study, a community survey, we were earnestly urged to take blood samples. It is important to note that this is a quite different issue from the problem of studying a population which is difficult to sample and for which non-random solutions have to be found, as in the pioneering Western Sydney Beats study (Bennett, Chapman and Bray, 1989a).

Second, there has been widespread inappropriate use of self-administered paper-and-pencil questionnaires; in such research the *meanings* of respondents' answers are completely unknown, being both unexamined and uncontrolled by the research procedures. This problem is compounded by the common practice of drawing conclusions from individual items in such questionnaires, where both validity and reliability are unchecked, and are probably poor. Paper-and-pencil tests have class and language biases which severely restrict the groups with which they can be used. From any methodological point of view, in an area as fraught with emotion, hypocrisy and threat as AIDS and sexuality, the self-administered paper-and-pencil questionnaire should be the *last* method one would choose, rather than the first.

Third, there has been much superficial analysis; a good many reports of quantitative studies show little beyond item-by-item frequency tabulations. Where cross-classifications are presented, there is often no clear rationale for the choice of variables to cross-classify. There is almost never a systematic examination of the patterns of relationships among and between groups of variables. This is not to say that more complicated statistics must be better — quite the contrary, the simpler the better, provided they do the job. It is to say that the findings of research are hardly ever interrogated with a view to answering questions about the social *processes* at work. Yet it is the social processes in the situation about which activists, educators and policy makers most need to know.

Fourth, there is the issue of obscure reporting; much of the research is reported in a language, or in places, that make it inaccessible to those workers who would in principle be its main users, and who could certainly give critical feedback. Worse, some research is reported in tiny fragments in scattered journals. This makes the researcher's publication list look lovely, but means that any user trying to understand the *pattern* of findings in a study has to search out and reassemble the fragments — which may not even be consistent when reassembled. Little collective thought has been given to how to make research accessible as well as useful.

Social science takes too little account of its communication practices. Sociology and economics in particular have reputations for jargon and obscurantism. We recognize good writers, but think of them as a kind of fluke. We teach our students how to crunch numbers but not how to build paragraphs. We ask them to reflect on social scientists' relationships with their 'subjects' but not on their relationships with their readers. Does it matter? The average readership of a paper in a scientific journal is remarkably small, so literary polish is hardly needed. But in an area like AIDS prevention, questions of communication do matter. It matters that the message is a useful one in the first place, that it gets out promptly, that it gets into the right hands, that it is accurately understood. The conventions of academic publishing are more likely to be a hindrance than a help with these goals. Yet academic publishing still matters, to provide for informed scrutiny, and to help future grant applications.

SAPA does have some useful lessons for a social science that will be more realistic, more sensitive to setting and social process, and more useful for a democratic, collective response to health issues. If SAPA has had any impact on the design of health research, we hope above all that it will be in encouraging a recognition of the *social*, the existence of collectivities and institutions, as a vital dimension in health research.

These technical weaknesses in current research can be remedied by means at hand. It is a question of lifting the quality of the survey research, and deploying a range of other research and analytic techniques such as participant observation, life-history studies, institutional research and deconstruction to complement the survey work. The more serious question concerns the conceptual agenda of HIV/AIDS research. Here two broad problems can be identified. First is the lack of concern with social setting and social process. It is not an accident that in the dominant discourse the social science contribution is translated as 'behavioural' research. The philosophical individualism that underpins much of mainstream medicine and psychology makes 'the individual' or the piece of 'behaviour' the basic unit of analysis. Combined with abstracted research methods, this produces an *elision of history and social process*. In popular discourses such as media talk about AIDS, the elided history is liable to be replaced by simplistic moral categories, such as the 'innocent victim' and the 'gay plague'. In policy discourse the process of elision results in categories such as 'behaviour change as an outcome of intervention programs', which effectively deny the agency, and especially the collective agency, of groups who are responding to the epidemic among them.

From such a perspective, questions of social dynamics and institutional processes hardly register. But these may be crucial in health issues. In mortality from gunshot, a crucial cause is the institutional availability of guns — witness California. With alcohol-related deaths and injuries on the roads, a crucial variable is the institutional and cultural availability of alcohol. The tremendous pressure of cultural dynamics such as institutionalized homophobia sometimes filters through in the AIDS research. But these dynamics cannot be properly understood unless they are directly studied, explicitly seen as the object of research. This is now happening in some US and UK research (Crimp, 1988; Fee and Fox, 1988; Watney, 1987).

To put all this in a formula, the level of *the social* needs to be re-inserted in the research in a constitutive way. Thus, for instance, the 'gay community' *as such* becomes a focus of research, reflection and analysis, not just the 'homosexual individual' or an aggregate of homosexual individuals. Similarly the networks of injecting drug users (one is less willing to speak of a 'community' here), and the underground industry that supports them, appear as a key object of knowledge. We need to research folkways, communication networks, the economics of drug use, sexual negotiation, etc. to grasp the capacities for sustainable change in this specific milieu.

The second problem is the top-down way in which the overall research agenda has been constructed. This is a little surprising given the number of gay men involved in the research effort. It is nonetheless true that the agenda has been constructed from an administrative rather than a community point of view. The questions it poses are principally those that arise from the standpoint of a medical administrator seeking to deploy the resources of the profession and the state to deal with the epidemic. How fast will the case load grow? Are advertising dollars effectively spent? Is mandatory testing justified? What is the next 'risk group'? A striking index of this is the amount of research that is concerned to define and distinguish 'target groups'. The language itself seems very revealing of a prevention strategy that presumes (a) an authoritative, knowledgeable, powerful centre, ready to fire its bullets of information or persuasion at identified targets; and (b) a dispersed, passive, ignorant periphery waiting to be fired at.

The dominant model of health education that has been adopted by many AIDS researchers, particularly in the United States, is a refinement of what might be called the KAP (or KAB) model — knowledge, attitudes, practices (or behaviour). The KAP model is a linear one, which initially assumed that knowledge shapes or determines attitudes which, in turn, shape or determine behaviour. In more recent formulations of the model, the theory of reasoned action (Ajzen and Fishbein, 1980; Ajzen and Madden, 1986) and the health belief model (Becker and Joseph, 1988), past behaviour is recognized as an important determinant of present behaviour, as are intention and subjective norms. The model has also been elaborated to include variables such as risk appraisal and personal susceptibility to harm (Weinstein, 1984) and self-efficacy (Bandura, 1989). Even with these refinements, the health effects or KAP model is still basically a linear one, the knowledge set of variables being seen as having an effect on the personality variables which then feed into behaviour, specifically into behavioural change. The model is used to set up interventions at various levels, that is, to provide communications about beliefs, attitudes, intentions and so on, which will eventually flow through to behavioural change, though it may be necessary to intervene at the second level by increasing perceptions of risk.

Even given its refinements and extensions, this is a poor model of education and an impoverished agenda for social research. One of the great accomplishments of contemporary social analysis — in theoretical developments mainly of the last two decades — is in developing ways of recognizing the *agency* of persons and groups without losing a grasp of the constraints of social structure (Harre, 1983; Giddens, 1984). Contemporary social science can feed into our understanding of health and medicine a much wider understanding of human social agency, its potentialities and limits, than has been possible before — and a very much richer understanding than anything in conventional models of 'health education' or 'behaviour change'.

A research agenda constructed from below, rather than from an administrative point of view, would be talking not about 'targeting' but about the various forms and occasions of collective self-help. The kinds of information most useful to that process may be substantially different from the kinds of information most interesting to administrators. For instance, this approach would give prominence to documenting *action models*, that is, examples of successful self-help activities, and not only in the AIDS field. It would certainly give much more attention to educational processes and dynamics; there is a worrying absence from the AIDS agenda of substantive and sophisticated educational research. It would give prominence to questions about how to change the functioning of institutions, such as hospitals, universities, schools. This is another absence from the current Australian AIDS research literature, except at the generalized level of discussions of policy formation.

We suggested at the beginning that social action is critical in dealing with the HIV epidemic and, in consequence, that social research should have a major role in policy formation. By and large it has not. The social sciences will gain a stronger voice and become more consistently useful, not by conforming more closely to the conventions of medical and biological research, but by conforming *less*. They need to pursue more boldly what is distinctively social in the issues surrounding HIV and AIDS, to have the courage of their own concepts and their own diversity of methods.

Perhaps what we most need is *more theory* — not in the form of cloudy abstractions but in the form of theory-at-work, careful dissection of problems and arguing of possible solutions. There are, for instance, some difficult questions about the social construction of sexuality embedded in the notion of gay 'identity'. Making progress with them might have very practical implications for the problem of entering and sustaining safe sex regimes.

Outline of the Book

We begin with an outline of the history of the Australian response to HIV and AIDS (Chapter 2). In Chapter 3 we describe the way the SAPA project developed and the context of the study. We also outline the design of the questionnaire and the rationale for the method. In Chapter 4 there is a detailed description of the fieldwork and a rationale for the development and use of the scales which became an important part of the analysis. In this chapter we describe the ways in which we recruited the men into the study and the sample of men who took part in the survey. In Chapter 5 we describe the sexual practices and preferences of the men in the study, and in Chapter 6 the correlates of sexual practice. These two chapters provide a backdrop for the discussion of changes in sexual practice which we describe in Chapter 7. Chapters 8 and 9 detail the ways in which informed social support and attachment to gay community shaped the adoption of safe sexual practices among the men. Chapter 10 discusses particular issues raised by bisexuality. In Chapter 11 we report on a follow-up survey, the Sustaining Safe Sex study, which we carried out four to five years after the SAPA survey. Chapter 12 integrates the findings of the two studies and outlines the prevention strategies which men in New South Wales have adopted in their response to HIV and AIDS. In this chapter we also refer to other research which was developed in the wake of SAPA.

Here we define some terms that we use in the book: the term 'safe sex' is used in preference to 'safer sex'; it is the term agreed by the Australian National Committee on AIDS, the national advisory body to the Australian government. The term 'safe sex' is used to refer to sexual activity, abstracted from the context of its enactment, that is currently deemed to be safe with regard to HIV transmission; for example, mutual masturbation is safe and anal intercourse with a condom is safe. The term 'unsafe sex' is used to refer to sexual activity, abstracted from the context of its enactment, that is currently deemed unsafe with regard to HIV transmission; for example, unprotected anal intercourse and fisting.

Chapter 2

AIDS in Australia

The first case of Acquired Immune Deficiency Syndrome (AIDS) was diagnosed in Australia in 1982 (Penny *et al.*, 1983). The human immunodeficiency virus (HIV) epidemic, as it came to be known, had begun. Health professionals, however, were only one of the 'expert' social groupings which came to affect the national response to the epidemic. By the time the mass media began to inform the general public of this new health threat, the gay communities were already aware of what was coming; they had been discussing the disturbing illnesses appearing among gay men in North America in their local gay newspapers and had been reading the overseas gay press. Australia's gay communities were well connected to their North American counterparts, and had for a long time been influenced by the politics and culture of the emergent modern gay communities in San Francisco and New York in particular. This 'Americanization of the homosexual' (Altman, 1982) flagged the significant expansion which took place among Sydney's highly visible gay community during the 1970s and 1980s. It was this Sydney community which was to be worst affected by the HIV epidemic.

By 1984 it was clear that Australia was going to experience a significant epidemic, and government public health machinery, after a faltering start in 1983, moved into top gear, establishing the institutional arrangements and policies which have guided the country since. It is important to recognize that from the start the country's response to the epidemic has involved three groupings: the Commonwealth, state and territory governments, and their public health officials; the non-government sector, initially and predominantly the gay communities' AIDS organizations; health professionals and research academics.

9

Table 2.1. AIDS by Sex and Exposure Category to 30 June 1992

Exposure category	Male	Female	Total	Percentage
Male-to-male sexual contact	2887	—	2887	85.7
Male-to-male sex and ID use	89	—	89	2.6
ID use (heterosexual)	38	28	66	2.0
Heterosexual contact	60	25	85	2.5
Haemophilia, etc.	49	0	49	1.5
Blood transfusion, etc.	62	39	101	3.0
Mother with HIV	4	4	8	0.2
Other/undetermined	71	8	83*	2.5
Total	3260	104	3368*	100.0

Note: * Persons whose sex was reported as transsexual are included here.
Source: Adapted from NCHECR (1992a).

AIDS Caseload

By 30 June 1992, 3368 cases of AIDS had been recorded in Australia, 66 per cent of whom had died (National Centre in HIV Epidemiology and Clinical Research [hereafter NCHECR], 1992a). Men account for 97 per cent of AIDS cases, and 1.3 per cent are under 20 years of age (see Table 2.1). The rate of increase in new AIDS diagnoses has slowed dramatically in recent years: 40 per cent in 1988, dropping to 6 per cent in 1991 (NCHECR, 1992a). Transmission mode categories used by Australian epidemiologists follow, in general, those of the United States Centers for Disease Control and the World Health Organisation's Global Programme of AIDS, although there is some debate as to the conceptual usefulness of these categories (Kippax, Crawford and Waldby, 1989).

This patterning of transmission would place Australia among *pattern one* countries, although this taxonomy is subject to considerable criticism (Patton, 1990), and in reference to Australia is somewhat misleading. The Australian epidemic has remained an epidemic of *sexual* transmission and one that is predominantly male-to-male sexual transmission (see Table 2.2), even though rates of increase in new diagnoses of AIDS related to male-to-male sexual transmission have slowed substantially in recent years, and cases of newly diagnosed AIDS related to haemophilia, heterosexual contact and those for whom no exposure category is available have recently increased (NCHECR, 1992b). This pattern is different from that found in the United States and most other Western countries and marks one of the basic differences between those countries and Australia.

To speak of an Australian epidemic is also misleading. New South Wales (NSW), the largest state, accounts for 62 per cent of national

Table 2.2. AIDS Cases by Exposure Category, 1982–1991

Exposure category	1982	1983	1984	1985	1986	1987	1988	1989	1990	1991
					(percentages)					
Male-to-male sexual contact	100.0	66.7	71.7	80.8	87.2	86.9	88.8	87.2	86.1	83.4
Male-to-male sex and IDU	0.0	33.3	2.2	0.8	4.8	2.1	3.0	2.6	1.6	3.1
IDU (heterosexual)	0.0	0.0	0.0	0.0	0.9	0.5	2.1	2.2	1.8	3.4
Heterosexual contact	0.0	0.0	0.0	0.8	0.0	1.6	1.5	1.4	3.0	3.8
Haemophilia, etc.	0.0	0.0	4.3	0.8	0.9	1.6	1.3	1.7	1.9	1.0
Transfusions, etc.	0.0	0.0	21.7	13.6	5.3	5.3	1.3	1.7	1.8	1.7
Mother with HIV	0.0	0.0	0.0	0.8	0.0	0.0	0.2	0.2	0.5	0.3
Other/undetermined	0.0	0.0	0.0	2.4	0.9	1.9	1.7	2.9	3.4	3.3

Source: Adapted from NCHECR (1992b, 1992c).

AIDS cases, and Sydney, its capital and the largest Australian city (population 3.5 million), accounts for over 55 per cent of the national AIDS total. Even this city-wide focus is misleading, as three inner-Sydney health districts, the Eastern, Central and Northern Sydney Area Health Services, together account for 48 per cent of the national AIDS total (New South Wales Health Department, 1990). Two of these inner-Sydney health districts take in the 'Oxford Street' quarter, the centre of Sydney's gay community and its social and commercial life.

HIV Infection

The overall level of HIV infection in Australia is harder to gauge. By 30 June 1992, 16,337 diagnoses of HIV infection had been recorded, 83 per cent of these in men (NCHECR, 1992a). It is estimated, however, that between 20,000 and 25,000 Australians could be infected (Solomon, Fazekas de St Groth and Wilson, 1990). NSW accounts for 67 per cent of the national HIV infection total.

Reported HIV infections increased by 1209 cases during the twelve months to 31 December 1991, an 8 per cent increase in the overall numbers of infected Australians (NCHECR, 1992a). The pattern of reported HIV infections, by exposure category, remains stable, and in 1991 these were substantially ascribed to male-to-male sexual contact (82 per cent). Other categories accounted for the following: male-to-male sexual contact and injecting drug use (3 per cent), injecting drug use among heterosexuals (5 per cent), heterosexual contact (5 per cent), haemophilia, etc. (3 per cent), blood transfusion, etc. (2 per cent), mother with HIV (0.2 per cent) (NCHECR, 1992a).

Homosexually Active Men and HIV/AIDS

To date, the Australian HIV epidemic has been and remains one over-whelmingly related to male-to-male sexual transmission of the virus, and the great majority of such infections has occurred among men in the identifiable gay communities. The earliest prospective study of HIV/AIDS among gay community identified men in inner Sydney found that 39 per cent of men were infected in 1985; this had risen to 49 per cent by 1987, but the rate of new infection had dropped from 8 per cent per annum to less than 0.5 per cent per annum (Burcham *et al.*, 1989). Recent research comparing data from this prospective study, an anonymous HIV antibody testing site in inner Sydney, and the blood-donor screening program indicates substantial decreases in the HIV seroconversion rate among homosexually active men (Kaldor *et al.*, 1991). Our own study on homosexually and bisexually active men in Sydney and parts of NSW, the Social Aspects of the Prevention of AIDS project (SAPA), based at Macquarie University, Sydney, found in the first survey in 1986–87 that 68 per cent of men had been tested, and of those 25 per cent were infected. Of the infected men, 76 per cent lived in the inner-Sydney area (Dowsett, Davis and Connell, 1992b).

These are not definitive figures for HIV seroprevalence among gay community identified men in Sydney, but are an indication of the intensity of the epidemic in that particular community. Estimated infection rates in gay communities in some other Australian cities are based on similar cross-sectional surveys and can only be regarded as a rough guide: 16 per cent in Melbourne (Campbell *et al.*, 1988); 7 per cent in Brisbane (Frazer *et al.*, 1988); 5 per cent in Canberra (Kippax *et al.*, 1989). While not all those infected through homosexual trans-mission are part of organized and recognizable gay communities in Australia, gay communities, and the inner-Sydney gay community in particular, were and continue to be the most affected social groupings in the country.

The National HIV/AIDS Strategy

Even though the expected dramatic increase among heterosexuals and injecting drug users has not occurred in Australia, there is no room for complacency. In the absence of evidence that infection rates via needle-sharing and heterosexual contact modes will not reach a 'take-off' point, the Australian response to the epidemic has been based on a strategy of careful monitoring of these possibilities. From 1984 onwards the Commonwealth government pursued a policy of cooperation and consultation with the affected communities, national medical bodies and other state and federal institutions, in order to create a unified national response. This policy was partly necessitated by Australia's federal system of government, for example, the states are wholly responsible for the delivery of health services, and partly by an initial recognition that the first affected communities, the gay communities, were already mobilized and informed about the problem and had taken their own steps to deal with it. It is important to remember that gay men first invented the idea and practices involved in 'safe sex' (Patton, 1989). Australian gay communities had already been developing preventive education materials in 1983 before any government assistance was provided, just as they developed the first volunteer care and support programs for people living with AIDS (Dowsett, 1989a).

Relations between the groupings involved in HIV/AIDS were patchy until late 1984 when the first fully developed national policies emerged (see Ballard, 1989). As government funds began to flow to the already active gay community-based AIDS service organizations and other non-government bodies, more systematic preventive education strategies and programs of care and support were developed. The volunteer-based, gay community AIDS Action Committees, established in each state in 1983 to lobby and provide the first education and care and support efforts within the gay communities, were transformed into AIDS Councils in 1985, and soon federated into the Australian Federation of AIDS Organizations (AFAO). (AFAO now also contains many other non-gay organizations, e.g., sex worker collectives and injecting drug users' self-help groups.)

A division of labour in preventive education was soon established: the Commonwealth government would retain responsibility for the national mass media education programs; the states would be largely responsible for health services delivery and some state-specific prevention activity, for example, schools programs; the non-governmental organizations would undertake the task of educating their affected communities. Similar specialization was to occur in care and support programs, for example, the national health scheme, Medicare, funds all hospital costs associated with HIV infection in Australia, but the gay community AIDS organizations would provide much of the volunteer home care for those infected with HIV or living with AIDS. Research, however, was to be funded separately through a special Commonwealth AIDS Research Grants Committee.

These arrangements mean considerable direct government funding of gay community-based agencies and programs, of injecting drug user groups, of sex worker collectives, of haemophilia organizations and so on. At times these funds are delivered directly to the non-government sector by the Commonwealth; however, most are dispersed via the state governments' HIV/AIDS units or bureaux in relationships marked in the main by a high degree of cooperation and mutual respect.

From 1984 until 1989 this policy evolved, with adjustments made to the mechanisms and the balance of representation of various interested groupings. Considerable increases in funding accompanied these policy developments. In 1990 the policy and its mechanisms for consultation and decision-making were definitively outlined in the *National HIV/ AIDS Strategy* (Commonwealth of Australia, 1989), designed to guide the country through the next three years. This national strategy was evaluated throughout 1992 and will be renewed by mid-1993.

The cooperative political and institutional arrangements for the Australian response to the epidemic are important to keep in mind when one assesses the programs of prevention undertaken among homosexually active men. While the relations between governments, health professionals and the community sector have often been difficult, even abrasive, and have led to direct political action on the part of gay communities at times, these arrangements allow for considerable flexibility in program management and delivery. In particular, the gay community AIDS organizations have been given significant funding and considerable liberty to undertake their own programs of prevention. The nation has listened to gay communities in this epidemic, and three states have decriminalized homosexual practices between men since 1985. Only one Australian state, Tasmania, has yet to do so. This is a very different situation from that in many parts of the United States or Great Britain.

Preventive Education among Homosexually Active Men

The gay communities of Australia rapidly developed their own early analysis of the HIV epidemic, its political setting and the emerging ideological positions of the actors, and pursued a remarkably astute response. Community-based educators of gay and bisexual men have developed substantial expertise in the last decade in devising and delivering educational programs on HIV/AIDS. The AIDS Councils did not come to HIV/AIDS work cold; many of their workers and volunteers had a long history of gay activism, and some earlier work in gay health had been occurring in the early 1980s. An annual conference on gay and lesbian health has been running for a number of years in the United States, and a concern with sexual health among gay men had been expressed in the Australian gay press since the late 1970s. The earliest news stories of the diseases which became AIDS were carried almost exclusively by the gay press in Australia until 1983–84, when patchy and often sensational coverage began in the mainstream press.

All but the most recent preventive education directed to gay men and other homosexually and bisexually active men has been developed and delivered by non-government organizations and almost always through gay community-based agencies. Although most, if not all, such programs were funded by government agencies, it was not until 1991, nine years after the first AIDS case in Australia, that preventive education campaigns directed to homosexually active men were designed and delivered by government bodies.

The preventive education strategies employed by gay community AIDS organizations involve much that is familiar in health promotion: information distribution through pamphlets, posters, newspaper advertisements; and information and support activities, usually involving group processes such as seminars, conferences and discussion nights. Gay community groups were able to rely on a culture of considerable and open discussion of sex among gay men. This facilitated an approach to education messages in image, style, language and meaning which could be sure of direct effect, particularly on gay-identified men. Many of these are shaped by the culture of the existing gay communities themselves. The institutions, organizations and commercial venues which constitute the infrastructure of the gay communities are utilized as distribution and reinforcement points in education.

A good example is the work done at politico-cultural events such as during the annual Sydney Gay and Lesbian Mardi Gras, a month-long festival culminating in a street parade watched by over 400,000 spectators and followed by an all-night dance party catering for over 17,000. During this period 'safe sex' campaigns are run, featuring specially designed posters and pamphlets, disco songs, video clips in gay community venues, and thousands of condoms are distributed in special flip-top packets. Floats in the parade, costumes and street theatre activities exhort gay men to practise 'safe sex' to protect themselves and their community. The Mid-Summa Festival in Melbourne offers a similar opportunity. In other cities comparable activities occur, focused on taking the message about HIV and 'safe sex' to gay men where they are, in whatever they do.

These community events become moments for educational campaigns which attempt to link gay men to a 'safe sex' culture, invoking the notion of a community acting to protect itself. Community leaders, entertainers and gay media are all involved. These can be termed *community intervention strategies*; they rely on inserting 'safe sex' information and other educational materials into the existing framework of gay community culture and its practices (Dowsett, 1990). They utilize existing cultural forms, institutions and practices as the vehicles for the transformation of behaviour. These are important strategies for they create a continuity with existing culture for 'safe sex' practices. They acknowledge, but also reduce, the dislocation caused by the epidemic in the lives of gay men. Such interventions also directly address those aspects of gay community life which were implicated in creating the environment for the male-to-male sexual transmission of HIV, such as sex-on-premises venues, events with considerable sexual activity and partner acquisition, 'beats' (places where men meet each other for casual sex, such as parks and public toilets) and so on. They modify a culture of sexual recreation and exploration to ensure that it is conducted safely.

These intervention strategies of the community educators have changed as the epidemic itself changed. During the early years the various print materials produced concentrated on the symptoms of HIV infection and a lengthening list of judgments about the safety of, or risk associated with, certain sexual practices. In the hands of the gay community AIDS organizations these print materials were a far cry from dry clinical lists of 'do's' and 'don'ts' of the sort typical, for a time, of government-produced materials. Increasingly, images and iconography from the gay communities themselves have shaped the form, tone and delivery of their educational materials and programs.

These more subculturally specific configurations of homosexual sex were (and are) controversial; at times they have raised the ire of Australia's more conservative powers-that-be and worried supporters within government and the public health bureaucracies. Debates continue over the use of homoerotic imagery, explicit language and the access of the 'general public', especially youth, to such information and representations of homosexuality. At times government funding has been withdrawn from specific materials. This is but one instance wherein the tense relationship between Australian society and its conspicuous homosexual communities underlies the response to HIV/AIDS.

Marshall (1990) argues that these pro-gay configurations are the only countervailing imagery available to gay men in the face of the mass media's representations of epidemic: 'innocent' versus 'guilty' 'victims'; photos of those ravaged by this 'killer' disease. As such, these pro-gay representations constitute another significant method of attaching gay community identified men to a collective project of stopping the epidemic.

The content of much of the education campaign material actually encodes and discloses a history of previous tumult and debate within the gay communities about the epidemic and its likely transmission routes, which took place in gay community media and activism from 1983 onward. Australia had its parallels to *How to Have Sex in an Epidemic* (Callen, 1983) and the anal sex debates in the United States (Shilts, 1988). The effects of this early gay community activity are detected in decreases in gonorrhoea observed among homosexual men from the early 1980s onwards, long before definitive HIV preventive education had occurred (Australian Gonococcal Surveillance Program, 1988; Donovan, 1988).

These *community intervention strategies*, as outlined above, posed problems for community educators: how to devise strategies for preventive education which relied less on gay iconography and reached those homosexually active men distanced from gay communities? To reach these men, often called the 'hard-to-reach', the gay community educators were by 1988 already developing programs which can be called *community attachment strategies* (Dowsett, 1990). These take the form of *peer* education programs, which differ markedly from state to state, but which in essence offer opportunities for men linked by age, or sexual interests, or region, to participate in programs of education about HIV and its transmission and to sustain safe sex (Davis, 1990; Parnell, 1992). Similar programs for men of Asian heritage, the hearing impaired, bisexually active men, and mature gay men are occurring. In addition, education programs for HIV-infected men have been developed. Many policy-makers erroneously consider those people living with HIV and AIDS in need of medical help only and fail to recognize the educational support and assistance HIV-infected people need in adapting their lives to the infection. (For a full description of these projects see AIDS Council of NSW, 1992.)

A second form of attachment program is the *outreach* project, such as telephone hotlines, supplying educational materials and condoms to suburban social networks and groups, and developing programs especially designed to educate men who use public places, 'beats', to meet other men for sex. Teams of educators regularly monitor the

17

activities of men at these places, distributing condoms, handing out pamphlets, and referring men to other programs and agencies if necessary (van Reyk, 1990; Davis, Klemmer and Dowsett, 1991). Originally this program started in Sydney, but similar projects are now operating throughout Australia (Dowsett and Davis, 1992).

While each project around Australia takes a slightly different form, all projects recognize that many men may not wish or be able to leave family, region, background, job and personal history to move to inner-city gay communities. For many, homosexual interests may be met more satisfactorily in clandestine and casual encounters than among the glitter of gay bars and discos. Increasingly, the patterning of homosexual interests by the effects of social class is becoming evident in the beats projects as well. There has been a remarkable development of new programs along these lines, and the AIDS councils continue to stretch their reach; yet it is clear that more remains to be done (O'Reilly, 1991).

These programs are developed by paid staff with volunteer workers, and the range of work has increased considerably over the past five years. By 1992 the largest of the gay community AIDS organizations, Sydney-based AIDS Council of NSW, had a full-time staff of over sixty and a number of other staff employed on fixed term projects. The AIDS Council of NSW has three branches and two regional offices in NSW and a total annual income of A$5 million. Until 1987, when the first of the national mass media HIV/AIDS prevention campaigns began, the AIDS Council of NSW was the only organization designing specific 'safe sex' educational programs for gay men in NSW.

We see in this brief history the development of the informal, collective gay community processes from 1980 onward to the later more systematic funded programs of prevention. The gay community agencies, with their intervention and attachment programs devised and delivered by paid staff and volunteers, many of whom are HIV-infected themselves, form the backbone of the Australian preventive response to HIV. The fact that all but the most recent programs directed at the prevention of homosexual transmission of the virus have been the product of gay community efforts means that Australia is extremely well placed to assess the impact of these prevention strategies on reducing the impact of the HIV epidemic among gay men and other homosexually and bisexually active men. As the SAPA project undertook its first large-scale survey in late 1986, before the first mass media prevention campaigns were undertaken in Australia, the project was in a good position to evaluate the effectiveness of these early gay community prevention efforts. Moreover, the direct and almost total control of this preventive education by the gay community-based AIDS organizations offered a unique opportunity to examine the impact of the gay communities themselves — not just as target audiences for education but as vehicles for producing change.

Chapter 3

The SAPA Project

The Social Aspects of the Prevention of AIDS (SAPA) project began in late 1985 with an approach by the AIDS Council of New South Wales to social scientists at Macquarie University, outlining the need for an information base for the AIDS Council's prevention work among gay and bisexual men. A research group formed, some plans were roughed out, a formal steering committee was set up, grant applications were drafted, and funding came through in early 1986. We were into the field in September 1986.

The initial plan was for three linked studies: Study A, a large cross-sectional survey of gay and bisexual men in the state of New South Wales (NSW) focusing on sexual practices; Study B, a life-history study, much more intensive but with smaller numbers; and Study C, a media content study that would examine the information that the men in the other two studies were receiving. Study C, after initial planning, became a casualty of funds and time. Study B continued, though more slowly and on a smaller scale than we had hoped, and will be discussed briefly later. Study A grew, in time and cost, until it almost took over the program. It proved to be so complex and the data so rich that we eventually had to put limits on the resources of time and energy it absorbed.

It is Study A — the cross-sectional survey — that is the major focus of this book, but it is by no means the whole story. Other research and outreach work in the area of HIV prevention has developed around the SAPA project, and our interests and activities as researchers have expanded and at times diverged. This further activity has had benefits for the SAPA project itself. It has stimulated us to look at our data in new ways and, in turn, the SAPA project has informed our other activities both intellectually and as a model of a research process which is responsive to pressures for realism and usefulness. At the same time, progress in SAPA studies was slowed by the mushrooming of activity around them. Before discussing the survey in detail, we describe the context in which the project and the research process developed.

Reflexive Character of the Research

It is a key feature of the enterprise that the AIDS Council of NSW did not just suggest and commission this research but has remained closely involved with it. The steering committee (which met every six weeks or so) included both academics and AIDS Council members. There was an overlap of membership and some researchers were members of the AIDS Council and members of the gay community, while others were not. The researchers were informed by the members of the AIDS Council, and the members of the AIDS Council and gay community were informed by the researchers. It was a two-way process; there was a great deal of give and take. The questionnaire development, the recruitment strategy, the selection of interviewers and the dissemination strategy all illustrate this process.

Development of the Questionnaire

At each stage of the survey we worked with the AIDS Council and gay community. The first task was to design a survey instrument, a questionnaire, that would provide the beginnings of an information base for the AIDS Council's educators. A series of consultations was held between members of the project's steering committee plus full-time staff and men active in HIV/AIDS education and gay community work, in an attempt to define major information needs of practitioners and appropriate ways of meeting them. To do this, the researchers needed an accurate and detailed knowledge not only of homosexual sexual activity but of the contexts of that activity. The researchers also needed an understanding of the salience of sexual activity to gay identity and the importance of community to homosexually active men. The AIDS Council members needed to have an understanding of the constraints which survey methodology would place on the information they wanted.

We brain-stormed with members of the gay community, we read gay porn, we talked about the sexual and emotional relations between men. We occasionally, at least at the outset, embarrassed each other, we debated and argued, we read or re-read the work of Altman (1979, 1982); Kinsey, Pomeroy and Martin (1948); Freud (1964b); and Weeks (1977, 1981, 1985), among others. We debated what should be included, what left out, how long or short the questionnaire should be, how questions should be worded, the flow of the questionnaire, what should go first or early in the questionnaire and what should go last. Instruments used in several Australian and United States studies of gay and bisexual men were examined and many of their items adapted, especially from Campbell *et al.* (1986) and Bennett and Petherbridge (1986). Drafts of sections prepared by individual members of the steering committee were examined by the whole group in workshops before being edited. After some months, the questionnaire was drafted, subjected to the scrutiny of the gay community and AIDS Council members, and then piloted. Results of trial interviews were fed back through the core group in an intensive final editing process. The production of the questionnaire thus rested on a dialogue between gay men active in the HIV/AIDS field and the survey researchers in the steering committee. We detail the contents of the questionnaire later in this chapter.

Development of Recruitment Strategy

The second stage in the survey was the recruitment of the sample. The goal of the research was to assist educational work designed to stop the spread of HIV through male-to-male sexual practice. For this purpose the group of concern was homosexually active men, those men involved in some homosexual practice during the last five years regardless of their identity or sexual orientation. We were also interested in the role of gay community in education and prevention. Our sample, we hoped, would include both gay community attached men, and men who were not attached to gay community, or only marginally so.

We defined eligible respondents as any 'men who had sex with men', whether they thought of themselves as gay, bisexual or heterosexual. In fact the large majority of our respondents described themselves as gay or homosexual, and reported having sex with men only. Nine per cent described themselves as bisexual or heterosexual and a slightly larger number (11 per cent) reported having at least some sexual activity with women as well as men (in the recent past).

There are two major problems in sampling such a population. One is finding the subjects; the other, given the nature of the issues, is obtaining a response. On the first problem, neither the size nor the whereabouts of the target population are known with any precision, though some informed guesses can be made. Using random sampling techniques via areas or electoral rolls, in conjunction with a screening question to identify members of our eligible population, is theoretically possible but impractical. The resources required would have been prohibitive.

At least equal to the problem of finding the representative sample is that of getting responses. AIDS has been accompanied by extensive media emotionalism. The nature of our questionnaire required very detailed information about sexual, especially homosexual, practices. The interviewing was undertaken shortly after the introduction in NSW of compulsory notification of all HIV antibody positive test results. Harsher measures against homosexual men and people infected by HIV were being canvassed at the time, and fears about confidentiality were widespread in the target groups. Under the circumstances the sample had to be based on volunteers. It was not a simple job to recruit them. The help of the AIDS Council and the gay community was essential to the success of this phase in the study.

Lacking a sampling frame, we had to build a non-random sample that would be informative about the population. The general approach was to 'snowball' from starting points where some of the population sought could certainly be reached — mainly gay venues and organizations, personal contacts and men responding to publicity (see below for details). Two main measures were taken to achieve representativeness: diversifying the starting points as widely as possible; and monitoring social characteristics of the sample during fieldwork so that corrections could be applied if necessary. Age, occupation, ethnicity, level of education and sexual preference (gay versus bisexual) were monitored for this purpose.

Interviewers

To maximize rapport as well as to develop the study as a reflexive enterprise of the gay community, it was decided to employ gay men, although not exclusively, as interviewers. The majority of interviewers were recruited from the gay community itself and trained in field procedures by the project. From applicants responding to advertisements, twenty-seven were selected for training and twenty-five were employed in the fieldwork. Interviews were also undertaken by members of the steering group. Selection of interviewers gave priority to previous experience in interviewing, related professional experience, knowledge of HIV/AIDS issues, ease of rapport and commitment to project goals. We also tried to establish some diversity of age and social background. We expected that respondents might have strong preferences as to who interviewed them, and indeed a majority expressed a preference for being interviewed by a gay man. Darrow *et al.* (1986) concluded, for an American sample of gay men in an HIV/AIDS study, that interviewer effects were slight, and this was also the impression we gained during fieldwork. Such effects are perhaps being overridden by the degree of motivation necessary to enter the study. The fieldwork used AIDS Council offices as well as university offices.

Dissemination Strategy

The reflexivity of our approach is evident in the reporting and dissemination of our results. No reports of findings were issued until the steering committee were satisfied with them. Over the last six years the project has fed results from many projects back to the AIDS Council regularly, especially to its full-time education and prevention workers; and it has had some significant impact on the strategies the AIDS Council has adopted, e.g., the issue of 'targeting' recipients of educational strategies, where SAPA findings argued against conventional views of a need for narrowly focused campaigns.

Our strategy of data collection and analysis meant that we reported our findings in large chunks of data at a time. We were extremely reluctant to rush out with quick analyses or to make announcements of isolated findings. We felt that the central meaning of our data would lie in the *relationships* that it showed, in the evidence of *process* that it provided. Therefore, it was worth taking the trouble to dig methodically and thoroughly, and argue through the problems of analysis and interpretation until they were resolved.

This approach had its costs. There was a constant demand for information to feed into prevention work; and we were sharply criticized for not publishing more and sooner. Moreover, our decision to publish first in a series of substantial reports to the AIDS Council of NSW, the community sector and other practitioners, rather than in short pieces in (even slower) academic journals, drew criticism from the academy. Some of this criticism was less than constructive. The thorough analysis of a large and complex data set cannot be rushed, and the job is not a matter of reading in the data and printing out a fistful of frequency tabulations. Our concern with accountability to the practitioners made it essential that we communicated with them in ways that did justice to the complexity of the material, without loss of clarity or accessibility.

Yet our approach had genuine problems. Interactive and exploratory data analysis is not readily funded, and we worked hand-to-mouth in this phase. Since the analysis was complex and slow, the data became more and more out-of-date. Our strategy of analysis and reporting was a source of debate within the research group and generated criticism from outside. But this process meant that our main reports were thorough and substantial, and that the interpretations represented a fully argued consensus within the research group.

In all the ways detailed above, we have tried to keep an organic connection between the researchers and the users of research and, more generally, between the researchers and the group being studied. In taking this approach we were of course taking a position on an issue of epistemology and methodology. Most medical research (and much of the natural sciences, though not all) makes a sharp distinction between the scientific observer and the object of observation. This distinction has long been controversial in the social sciences, where a methodological tradition has developed which emphasizes the *reflexive* character of research as social or collective self-knowledge. Gagnon (1988) argues persuasively that there is much to be gained from blurring the distinction, e.g., by employing members of the group to be studied as co-researchers. Like Wadsworth (1987), we consider that research *designed* as participatory and reflexive is particularly appropriate in supporting community action — and it is, above all, community action that is needed to stop the spread of HIV. In SAPA the circuit of reflection was more complex than in most of the community initiatives discussed by Wadsworth; but we built in a process of accountability to the community which we think was reasonably successful in controlling any drift towards abstractness.

The problem often raised about reflexive research is that of 'objectivity': does this approach involve biased observation and reporting? Part of the answer is that it is meant to: we hoped to build in a bias towards practicality. But in terms of skewing the findings, of misrepresenting the actual state of affairs, reflexive research is in no more trouble than abstracted observation is. 'Objectivity', as Deutscher (1983) has argued in an important review of the term, is not a question of emotional distance. Enquiry is, indeed, predicated on an involvement sufficient to drive an attempt to understand fully. An *accurate understanding* of the problem being researched is more likely when one is self-conscious about one's own specific relationship to the problem than when all relationships are blurred under a single formula of abstraction.

Focus on Practice

As well as adopting a policy on reflexivity, we decided to focus our research on *practice*. Here we were guided by theoretical concerns. As noted in Chapter 1, health promotion research often takes the form of surveys of 'knowledge, attitudes and beliefs': characteristically paper-and-pencil questionnaires containing opinion or attitude scales, particulate tests of knowledge, and single-item self-reports of specific behaviours. Such research, derived from a particular American tradition of social psychology, is closely linked to individualistic models of health promotion and behaviour change. SAPA had some overlap with this genre — we included some attitude items — but the basic design of our questionnaire and the focus of our analysis were very different.

We thought it vital to move beyond the naive individualism of the literature on health behaviour change, to bring collectivities and social dynamics into view. At a logical level, personal action or practice is always predicated on social structure, and at the same time constitutes social structure (Giddens, 1984; Secord, 1982). In the HIV epidemic we are dealing much of the time with sexuality, and sexuality is socially constructed, relational, situational and culturally specific (Gagnon and Simon, 1974; Caplan, 1987).

Accordingly the basic concept on which the questionnaire was constructed is that of *social practice*. We sought, in great and even wearying detail, descriptions of what people actually do and have done, rather than opinions about what they ought to do or would like to do. We sought evidence of whole patterns of action, not just isolated behaviours. We sought evidence about the settings of interaction: for instance, always asking about given sexual practices in the context of a specific type of relationship; and asking a series of questions about participation in different aspects of gay social life. We explored types of relationships and transactions (for example, negotiations about condom use) in some detail.

Thus the interviews and later the analysis, built up a detailed picture of the respondents' sexuality, not as a set of individual behaviours, not even as behaviours-in-social-context, but as *social practice* per se, as the mutual constitution of personal and social life. As the analysis proceeded, the epistemological consequences of our research strategy became

27

apparent. A double object of knowledge appeared: on the one hand the *person* as social actor, on the other hand the *collectivity*, gay community. We were able to characterize the collectivity in certain ways, state some of the cultural dynamics operating in it, and make proposals about directions for collective action by this community.

There is also a severely practical point. An educational strategy (as distinct from a coercive strategy) for preventing the further spread of HIV must operate at the intersection between the physical action through which the virus is transmitted, and the 'meanings' through which the action is apprehended and experienced and through which it can, therefore, be reshaped. These meanings are not idiosyncratic. There is overwhelming evidence (see, for example, Gagnon and Simon, 1974) that sexual meanings are socially patterned, contextual, in a very strong sense. The focus on practice, then, is the theoretical means by which the practical problems of an educational strategy can be unravelled.

The SAPA Questionnaire

The cross-sectional survey which we called SAPA Study A used a very detailed forced-choice questionnaire to interview a moderately large sample (n = 535) of homosexually active men. The intention was to 'map' sexual practices and their social contexts and correlates. The questionnaire was long (fifty-eight pages covering nearly 1000 items of information) and inevitably complex, yet it worked well in the field and seems to have had few ambiguities. Its major sections, in order of administration, were:

a   personal and social descriptors (forty-eight items);
b   sexual identity (thirty-seven items);
c   gay community and social involvement (fifty-seven items);
d   sexual practice — enjoyment, frequency (regular and casual partners), sexual history (221 items);
e   media exposure, general AIDS knowledge and attitudes (ninety-two items);
f   safe sex knowledge and practice, changes in sexual practice, condoms (193 items);
g   sex with women (125 items);
h   prostitution (seventy-two items);
i   health practices, drugs, testing, relationship to people with AIDS (105 items);

j specific items for the Australian Capital Territory subsample (forty-one items).

Sample Definition and Recruitment

The approach to sampling was broadly in the Kinsey tradition, though where Kinsey, Pomeroy and Martin (1948) sought statistical *norms* for conceptually isolated behaviours, we mainly sought statistical *relationships* and evidence of social processes. The sampling method used is adequate for this purpose if a reasonable degree of diversity is achieved. A key question was how far we would succeed in reaching beyond 'Oxford Street' in inner Sydney.

Volunteers were sought by several means. One was, an appeal was issued through mainstream mass media. Media releases led to a number of radio interviews by members of the core group, and some newspaper articles, in which the study was described and volunteers invited to 'phone in. Advertisements were placed in certain regional newspapers. Another was advertising and stories in the gay press and on gay radio. A series of reports and interviews appeared during the fieldwork. We thought this particularly important to reach 'closeted' men who might use these media for personal-contact advertisements but not join openly gay groups. Thirdly, cards were distributed inviting participation, at clinics, venues, gay community functions, etc. Some 20,000 cards were distributed, a considerable proportion by hand in the course of visits to venues (hotels, discos, saunas, etc., a total of seventeen) and events (including nine Mardi Gras events) by project staff. This was combined with publicity in drag shows (we appreciate the performers' help), a stall at the Polympics (an annual gay sports day), and as much face-to-face publicity as we could contrive. The cards functioned mainly as background advertising; personal discussions proved the most effective way of recruiting volunteers. Fourthly, circulars were issued and visits paid to gay men's groups and organizations covering a wide range of activities — social, sporting, motoring, health, etc. They were also sent to all groups known to us through the AIDS Council of NSW, or through contact lists in the gay press (generally out-of-date), or who could be found by detective work and vigorous networking, were circularized. The SAPA Study A coordinator or an interviewer visited a considerable number, spoke to members and took bookings on the spot. Forty-seven groups were contacted in one or other of these ways. Fifth, personal networks were used. All respondents were asked to recruit further volunteers, and many did. Some known networks (especially in extra-metropolitan areas) were contacted and invited to participate. Finally, the interviewers themselves were considered as contact persons, and some spent time recruiting among their own networks (though not interviewing people known to them). Chapter 4 provides a detailed account of the sample and method.

Chapter 4

Method

With the questionnaire piloted, the recruitment of men underway and the interviewers trained (as described in Chapter 3), a fieldwork co-ordinator was appointed and the interviewing began.

Because of the highly sensitive nature of the data, the respondents were guaranteed anonymity, unless they chose otherwise. No names or contact addresses or telephone numbers were taken unless the men volunteered them, and only the senior researchers could match the names to the data. The men who volunteered their names were contacted again in 1991 as described in Chapter 11.

The recruitment strategy for the SAPA survey therefore relied upon men contacting the research team. Except where bookings were taken during a visit to a club or venue, respondents volunteered by telephoning the project, with a booking usually being made immediately. This allowed the respondent to control the contact (important in the circumstances already described) and minimized our problems of scheduling (severe in any case). It also constituted a distinct 'barrier to entry' into the sample, which had both good and bad consequences. On the good side was the high motivation of those who were interviewed. Despite the emotional difficulty of much of the questionnaire, very few interviews, once begun, were not completed. Most respondents answered carefully and appeared to be taking trouble to give an accurate account of their lives. This is one of the reasons we consider the data are of high quality relative to most survey research. On the other side, it probably restricted the sample in certain ways, for example, limiting the participation of people who did not have easy access to a telephone in conditions of privacy.

Four hundred and eighteen interviews were completed in the Sydney metropolitan area (as defined in Appendix 3: including Blue Mountains). One hundred and seventeen were completed in other parts of NSW and the ACT. The extra-metropolitan sample ranged from regional cities through country towns to the countryside, and included areas in the south, mid-west and north of the state. Contact was generally more difficult, and fieldwork costs (travelling expenses and wages per interview) much higher, outside the metropolitan area. Nevertheless, we thought this important both for the general analysis of the data (increasing the diversity of the sample in a major way) and for the specific issues around HIV/AIDS that arise for men in the country and in smaller cities.

Fieldwork began in mid-September 1986 and finished in early March 1987, with a lull in the holiday period of December-January. Some changes in recruitment methods were made over this period. The initial phase of mass media publicity saw 229 interviews completed by the end of October. In the second phase emphasis was given to personal networking and visits to organizations; another 191 interviews were completed in November-December. Monitoring of the questionnaires as they were returned had shown low numbers of working-class men and men born in non English-speaking countries; accordingly, in a third recruitment phase emphasis was given to publicity in western Sydney. One hundred and fifteen interviews were completed in January–March.

The characteristics of the sample on some of our monitoring variables changed a little, but on the whole remained impressively stable through the different stages of fieldwork. (The average level of education fell and there were more Australian-born in the final 200 interviews; but these changes were slight. Sexual preference, average age and labour force status remained constant.) Sample construction, therefore, was reasonably consistent over the full period of fieldwork.

Characteristics of Respondents

A simple tabulation of the personal and social characteristics of respondents minimally provided a 'profile' of the group whose sexuality and social life will be discussed later. Comparing these distributions with population distributions also provided an indication of what had happened in the sampling. We give detailed information about the nature of the sample in Appendix 2.

The difficulty in sampling this population is knowing what is the relevant population base, since gay and bisexual men and, more generally, homosexually active men do not constitute a category counted by the Australian Bureau of Statistics (ABS). Official statistics in any case have varying geographical and population coverage. The comparisons in Appendix 2 therefore have varying bases, though in all cases pertinent ones. Our ideal base for most purposes was 'NSW adult men in November 1986'. It was anticipated that our field methods, however careful, would not yield a perfect fit. What is know about the spread and incidence of sexual behaviour between men in our society suggests that the group being studied would in any case show some divergences from overall population averages.

The major conclusion that emerged from the data in Appendix 2 was that the social profile of the SAPA sample was not very exceptional or unusual. Across a range of variables the characteristics of respondents resembled, to a fair approximation, those of the general population of adult men. Where departures from population patterns occurred, they were generally consistent with each other and made good sense. Marked departures from general population patterns mostly occurred on items with obvious connections to the definition of the sample in terms of sexual practice: marital status, parenthood and to a lesser extent religion. Overall, we were more impressed with the social 'normality' of this sample than by its 'difference'. Though this is an atmospheric rather than a statistical judgement, we think it important to register in the face of stereotypes which emphasize the difference of homosexual men.

On the other hand some conventional ideas about gay men have a foundation in fact that was reflected in the sample. One was area of residence. It is apparent that some areas had substantially higher concentrations of gay men (for example, around Oxford Street and the inner-western suburbs) than others. Another concerned age. Freedom to have homosexual sex or become involved in male-male relationships can be expected to have had some connection with economic security and the age at which people leave the parental home. The age profile of a homosexual sample was also likely to reflect generational experience with the changing social attitudes toward homosexuality and therefore self-perceptions of homosexuality, depending on whether people grew up in the very repressive 1950s or the relatively open 1970s.

The study's sampling goal of diversity, ensuring both gay men as well as homosexually active men who were not part of gay community, was certainly reached. The metropolitan sample probably reflects reasonably well the geographical patterning of gay social life in Sydney. We noted above that the major goal of sampling was enough diversity to permit analysis of relationships, rather than an attempt to define parameters. On all the major social variables of concern, except the special case of ethnicity, there was enough diversity in the sample to make feasible correlational analysis or analysis of variance. Further, checks against general population distributions for social descriptors gave us some confidence that the measures of practice in the questionnaire, for which no direct population checks were possible, would not produce seriously unrepresentative results. We judge that the findings of the study should be reasonable approximations of what was happening in at least a large proportion of the gay and bisexual male population.

The major qualification to this judgment is in relation to social class. There was a clear underrepresentation of working-class men in the SAPA study, as evidenced by the distributions of occupation, education and to some extent place of residence (specifically, western Sydney). This is a common finding in research with samples of gay men both pre- and post-AIDS. For instance, a four-country sample from the late 1970s based on homosexual clubs has high educational levels and appears to have a low working-class component (Ross, 1986); the 1984 Adelaide prospective study on AIDS has 52 per cent tertiary-educated (Ross, 1986); the 1984–85 Chicago Multicenter AIDS Cohort Study (medical and psychosocial) reports a 'well-educated' sample (Joseph *et al.*, 1987); the 1984 telephone survey of gay men in San Francisco reports 88 per cent with at least some college education (Research and Decisions Corporation, 1984); a 1985 New York City study with a sampling strategy reasonably similar to SAPA reports remarkably high levels of education, with three-quarters having four or more years at college (Bauman and Siegel, 1987). The venue-based Melbourne study by the Victorian AIDS Council (Sinnott and Todd, 1988), conducted at around the same time as SAPA, also had high levels of education in Australian terms (see Appendix 2).

There are two obvious explanations: artefact of method, or characteristics of the population. Volunteer-based studies generally attract samples biased toward the higher educated and the more professionally employed, regardless of the sexual orientation of the subjects or the topic of research. This effect may well be exacerbated by the atmosphere of threat around the AIDS issue. Those coming forward were likely to be those with the most social resources to resist threat. On the other hand the population of gay men may genuinely differ from norms for heterosexual men in terms of education and occupation.

While male homosexual activity undoubtedly occurs throughout the occupational and class spectrum, research in Germany (Reiche and Dannecker, 1977) suggests that men who recognize their homosexuality are more inclined to move into some parts of the workforce than other parts. Relative levels of hostility or acceptance are likely to explain this phenomenon. The tendency is to move away from the manual or so-called 'blue-collar' occupations towards the tertiary or service sector of the economy, 'white collar' jobs, etc. There may also be educational effects. The universities have been a major base for gay liberation politics, and it is possible that the more tolerant atmosphere in institutions of higher education has made the formation of an openly homosexual identity more feasible among students than in other milieux.

It is also possible that these two explanations interact. What is known of the dynamics and development of sexual object choice gives little reason to think initial homosexual *preference* is any less common among working-class men. But what is known of social class suggests that the choice will find different patterns of *expression*. And it is the social realization of sexuality that encounters the communication processes of research.

This point applies also to the ethnic composition of the sample. Underrepresentation of men born in non English-speaking countries is to be expected in an English-language survey. But we think there is something more. Sexual practice and sexual relationships are constructed in different ways in different cultures. In particular there is reason to think the social acceptance of, or taboo against, homosexual activity differs a good deal between ethnic groups, perhaps more than actual sexual practices differ.

Data Analysis

The philosophy underlying the data analysis in the SAPA study is one in which the design of the questionnaire is integral to the data analysis. That is, the design of the questionnaire dictates the analyses that will be carried out. In turn, the theory underlying the data collection dictates the design of the questionnaire.

The theoretical basis for the SAPA study, as outlined above, was a social theory which stressed the importance of practice and its social context, and recognized that a community defines and is defined by a set of practices. It also recognizes that individuals and community interact in complex ways, that practices are multiply determined, and that what individuals do is influenced by structural variables. As discussed in Chapter 1, the model underlying the SAPA study is more complex and more realistic than traditional KAB or KAP (knowledge, attitudes, behaviours, practices) models which underlie many survey studies in the HIV/AIDS prevention area.

As mentioned above, in the SAPA study a large amount of information, almost 1000 individual items, was collected from each respondent. These items were not, however, randomly selected. The information collected fell into a number of areas or clusters, as suggested by the broad outline of the social theory referred to above. Thus there were a number of items of demographic information, namely age, education, income, employment status, occupation, country of birth, religion, which are referred to as structural variables in the various chapters of this book. A further set of variables is referred to as 'milieu' variables. These defined the particular social context in which the men lived. They include place of residence, type of sexual relationship, sexual identity, involvement in various gay community organizations, information about friends, contact with the HIV epidemic. Most of the remaining variables were designed to investigate patterns of sexual practice, sexual enjoyment, knowledge of safety of various sexual practices, knowledge and opinions about HIV/AIDS, responses to the HIV/AIDS epidemic, testing.

Data analysis proceeded in stages, beginning with an examination of patterns of relationships within the various sets or clusters of variables. At this stage, stable, reliable and meaningful indices were developed for the structural and milieu variables. At the next stage, the variables of central interest were examined. These included such things as knowledge of HIV transmission, knowledge of safe sexual practices, knowledge of unsafe sexual practices, patterns of sexual practice, enjoyment of sexual acts, patterns of response to the HIV/AIDS epidemic, and patterns of engagement with a gay community. In the analysis of these sections of the questionnaire, a number of 'scales' were developed.

Scale Development

A scale is a measure derived from individual items by assigning a numerical value to the response to each item in a consistent fashion and then combining the responses by adding the numerical values to form a score. Why would one want to do this? First of all, if the procedure just described is justified on statistical grounds (to be described below), the single score is then a meaningful summary of a number of individual items of information, thus providing a way of reporting a large amount of information in summary form.

Second, a score made up by combining items will be more reliable than any single item of information. Reliability, or rather unreliability, refers to the tendency for responses to questionnaire items to vary from one occasion to another. For example, suppose you ask someone in a survey to rate oral-genital sex with respect to risk of transmission of HIV, and the response categories are 'very safe', 'small risk' or 'not at all safe'. If an individual is not sure of the risk, he may be undecided about whether to respond 'very safe' or 'small risk'. On one occasion, say today, he may respond 'small risk', whereas tomorrow, when asked the same question, he may respond 'very safe'. This is unreliability. It can be shown that if items in a set are all measuring (to some extent at least) the same thing, then the combined score will be much more reliable than the score on any single item. The more items that can be combined, the more reliable is the score.

Third, the scale score provides a range of values across the sample, giving a large number of categories into which individuals may be categorized, and these categories are ordered. Each individual will have a score, and those with high scores may be assumed to differ from those with low scores as far as that characteristic is concerned. The scores on the scale may be used in data analysis procedures requiring a numerical level of measurement. For example, if one were endeavouring to measure 'knowledge of HIV transmission', a single item would divide the sample into two categories, those with the correct response and those with the incorrect response. A set of ten such items would give each individual a score from 0 to 10, distinguishing those with an extremely high score from those with a slightly lower score and so on. Analyzing 'knowledge of HIV transmission' in the latter case would enable a comparison of mean or average knowledge scores across age groups, income groups, education groups, rural versus urban and so on. Such an analysis is much more meaningful than an analysis limited to examining ten different items across the structural variables. Combining items, however, may be carried out only if certain conditions are satisfied by the data.

The Process of Scaling

A scale analysis is a procedure which assesses whether it is justifiable to combine a set of items into a single scale. It provides information about how good the scale is according to the criterion of how well the items belong together in a statistical sense.

Formal scale analysis works on the numerical properties of the data. In addition to satisfying the numerical criteria, the items to be combined must be a set of items which are conceptually similar and, in the case of a survey, were included in the questionnaire for the purpose of measuring one aspect of an indicator. Thus scale analysis is in a certain sense an hypothesis testing procedure.

We test theoretical assumptions (such as the assumptions of patterns of 'insertive' and 'receptive' sexual practice) by examining the pattern of correlations between pairs of items. In carrying out scale analysis and scale construction, we examine a number of items at a time. We take a set of items (for example, all items of insertive sexual practice) and look at the correlations between each pair of items. If all pairs of items are positively associated, that is, all correlations are positive, this is evidence that all of the items in the set of items are to some extent measuring the same thing. It is then possible to combine them into a single score, called a scale score.

The scale analysis also provides information on internal consistency of the scales (Cronbach's alpha or the coefficient of internal consistency). The coefficient of internal consistency is a statistic which ranges in value from 0 to 1. The closer it is to 1, the more confident we are in the proposition that the set of items is measuring a single entity. Values between 0.7 and 0.9 are usually regarded as fairly strong evidence that the scale can be justified.

Beyond Scaling: Factor Analysis

In a number of different areas in the SAPA study we used factor analysis to investigate the pattern of correlations found in the data. This was used, in particular, in those cases where hypotheses that items would be related to one another in particular ways (thus justifying certain scales) were not supported.

Factor analysis is related to scale analysis both theoretically and mathematically. When used in analyzing data from surveys, factor analysis, like scale analysis, starts with the correlations between pairs of items. Where it is believed that a set of items is measuring more than one thing in common, factor analysis is a way of examining the pattern of correlations to see how many different entities or constructs the items are measuring, and suggesting which items 'go together' to measure each construct. Identification of the constructs is then done by examining the content of the items which form each one. Thus this form of factor analysis (exploratory factor analysis) does not have the rigour of hypothesis testing found in scale analysis and in a more theoretically driven factor analysis procedure (confirmatory factor analysis).

Nevertheless, exploratory factor analysis is useful in areas where theory is lacking, and in exploratory and ground-breaking studies such as the investigation of male-to-male sexual practice carried out in the SAPA study. Here again, however, caution is needed. The items submitted to a factor analysis should be from the same conceptual domain. Although sexual practice of a certain kind may be correlated with education, it would be totally inappropriate to include education as an item in a factor analysis of sexual practice.

Having carried out a factor analysis, the results may not be clear-cut. The way we have used factor analysis is that the results of the factor analysis are examined to see whether there is strong evidence for the presence of one, two, three or more constructs in the set of items. Only if the items can be divided into separate sets do we then proceed, that is, when the constructs may be considered to be separate constructs, with no items which have a strong presence in more than one construct. Each set of items is then regarded as a candidate for a scale, and a scale analysis is carried out to investigate the properties of the scale. An example of factor analysis which resulted in three separate scales was a factor analysis of the items relating to sexual practice (see Chapter 5). If no clear and separable constructs appear as a result of the factor analysis, the set of items is not combined in any way.

Validity of Scale Scores

As well as being reliable and internally consistent, it is important that a scale score can be used as an indicator of a meaningful construct, that is, that the scale is a valid scale. To some extent the construction of the scale out of a set of items originally included in order to measure the construct concerned helps to ensure that the scale is valid. Some of the scales in the SAPA study, as already mentioned, were constructed from sets of items of this kind. Other scales were constructed out of sets of items from a particular domain where factor analysis was needed to suggest which items should be combined.

It is possible to examine whether the scale scores are valid indicators of theoretical (abstract) constructs by examining the way in which the scale scores are related to other items in the questionnaire. Thus the statistical analyses carried out using scale scores help to validate such scores as indicators of underlying theoretical constructs. For example, one would expect that, on average, men who live in the inner-Sydney area, the heart of the Sydney gay community, would have relatively high scores on the GCI (Gay Community Involvement) scale; that is, a statistical analysis (ANOVA) of GCI scores by locale would find a significantly higher mean GCI score for those in the inner-Sydney region. If this did not happen, it would throw doubt on the validity of the GCI scale as an indicator of Gay Community Involvement.

Using Scale Scores

Once the scales are developed, and their reliability and validity checked, scale scores can be used in statistical analyses to test hypotheses and investigate relationships in the data. Most of the analyses we carried out examined the relationship between scale scores and other key variables such as structural variables, milieu variables and variables concerned with the HIV/AIDS epidemic. For two key variables, we examined interrelationships between variables by means of multiple regression analyses. These two variables were scale scores, one the AS (Adoption of Safe sex) scale score and the other the RC (Relationship Change) scale score.

In carrying out the multiple regressions, we once again designed the analyses on theoretical grounds. The method used was a hierarchical regression modelling approach, examining the variables in 'families'. Using our approach to regression modelling, we were able to examine the importance of structural variables as predictors of change scores, the importance of milieu variables over and above structural variables, and the importance of things like knowledge of safe sex, knowledge of unsafe sex, and contact with the epidemic. These analyses are reported in Chapter 7.

Description of Scales

Here we describe the various scales we developed; technical details of these scales are given in Appendix 5.

1 Knowledge scales. Four knowledge scales emerged from the data: Knowledge of Safe Sex (KSS), Knowledge of Unsafe Sex (KUS), Knowledge of Social Practices (KSP), and General Issues (GI). In carrying out the scale analysis procedures, we found that we needed two scales to examine knowledge regarding the safety of sexual practices.

It was one of the unexpected findings of the study that accurate knowledge of safe sexual practices was negatively correlated with accurate knowledge of unsafe sexual practices. That is, a person with a high score for accuracy of knowledge of safe sexual practices was likely to have a *low* score for accuracy of knowledge of unsafe sexual practices. This unexpected result reflects the problematic nature of 'knowledge'. It is not a unitary concept, and people answer questions about what is 'safe' not only in accordance with what educational messages have been provided, but also in accordance with their own hopes, fears, experiences, beliefs and so on (see Chapter 8 for a full discussion).

The GI (General Issues) scale was also found to represent attitudes of caution or 'rashness', rather than 'knowledge'. It consisted of items such as 'It is unlikely that there will soon be a cure for AIDS' (where the responses from Strongly Agree to Strongly Disagree were scored from 1 to 5).

The KSP (Knowledge of Social Practices) scale measured the accuracy of knowledge that a number of common social practices, such as sharing a glass or spoon, are 'safe with regard to passing on the AIDS virus'.

2 Sources of knowledge scale. A scale of Pamphlet Awareness (PA) was constructed to measure the number of different sources of HIV/AIDS information that people reported having seen and/or read.

3 Sexual practice scales. The sexual practices were subjected to a factor analysis in order to examine meaningful patterns of sexual practice. The analysis of sexual practices is described in more detail in Chapter 5. As indicated above, three scales emerged from the analysis of patterns of sexual practice: an Oral Tactile Practices (OTP) scale, the scores on which represent the number of different oral/tactile practices a person engaged in; and an Essentially Anal Practices (EAP) scale, the scores on which represent the number of different anal practices a person engaged in; and a third scale of Infrequent Esoteric Practices (IEP), the scores on which represent the number of these practices a person engaged in. Most of our sample had scores of zero on this last scale.

4 Gay community attachment scales. Three scales were found necessary to represent different patterns of attachment to and engagement in gay community: Gay Community Involvement (GCI), Sexual Engagement in gay community (SXE) and Social Engagement in gay community (SCE).

The Gay Community Involvement (GCI) scale score is concerned with a political and cultural involvement in gay community. The items which make up the scale relate to organized gay activities as opposed to less formal social settings covered by the SCE scale. A key item in this scale is 'Do you see yourself personally as being part of the gay community?' This scale examines membership and activity in gay community organizations and culture.

The Sexual Engagement (SXE) scale score represents the breadth of sexual engagement: the number of casual partners, number of different places where sex is sought, and to some extent the number of different places where sex is practised.

The Social Engagement (SCE) scale score represents the extent to which the person's social life is lived in the company of gay male friends. It includes information about number of gay male friends, how much free time is spent with such men, number of different places where men go out with gay male friends.

It is important to note that these three scales were positively correlated to one another, that is, the concepts they are measuring overlap to some extent.

5 *Gay identity disclosure scale.* Gay Identity Disclosure (GID) related to the number of different categories of people to whom the respondent had disclosed his gay identity.

6 *Contact with the epidemic.* This scale (CE) consisted of only three items and indicated in a crude way the degree of contact with the epidemic.

7 *Change scales.* Two scales of key importance in our research were developed to measure the extent of change in the sexual lives of the men in our sample as a result of 'awareness of AIDS'. The first of these we named Relationship Change (RC). This scale consisted of the number of different changes to the pattern of sexual *relations* and *relationships* that a person said he had made as a result of 'awareness of AIDS'. Each item in this scale (see Appendix 5 for details) related to a reported change in the kind and/or number of sexual partners and the places where sexual partners were sought.

The second change scale was named AS (Adoption of Safe sex). Scores on this scale represent the number of different changes in sexual *behaviour* as a result of 'awareness of AIDS'. Items on this scale included, for example, 'masturbating alone' and 'using condoms'.

On both scales scores ranged from 1 to 4 according to whether the response category was 'I've stopped doing it', 'I'm doing it less', 'I'm doing it about the same (including never done it)', 'I've started doing it/I'm doing it more'.

Conclusion

Our research is described in some detail in the following chapters. We use scores on the scales described above as variables which may be analyzed by examining how they relate to each other as well as other structural and milieu variables. For example, are there differences in KSS scores according to place of residence? Is there a differences between HIV positive and HIV negative men in terms of EAP scores? Can we explain variation in AS scores as a function of CE scores? Of necessity, we use the scale scores in the numerical data analyses. In discussing our results, however, and in testing, modifying and building theory out of our data analysis, we are concerned to emphasize the underlying conceptual entities of which the scale scores are indicators — sometimes only crude indicators. One advantage of a well designed questionnaire is that it is possible to summarize information in a meaningful way by the construction of reliable and valid scales.

Chapter 5

The Picture of Sexuality

In the early days of modern sexology, as human sexual activity came under 'scientific' scrutiny, there was considerable interest in the social context of sexuality and in the way sexuality served as an arena of social relations. Krafft-Ebing's (1965) cases repeatedly documented social class relations in sexuality, a theme that deeply interested other Victorian commentators too (Marcuse, 1955). Freud's (1964a, 1964b) famous account of the shaping of sexuality through the life history connected sexuality closely with what we would now call the gender relations of the nuclear family.

However, the rise of a more positivist sexology during the twentieth century tended to untie 'sexual behaviour' from its social moorings. The great Kinsey studies (Kinsey, Pomeroy and Martin, 1948; Kinsey et al., 1953) abstracted orgasm from its meanings to produce a quantifiable unit of behaviour. Masters and Johnson (1966) even more sharply separated 'sexual response' as a matter of physiology from social relations.

There has been a significant reaction from this trend, a reassertion of the social character of human sexuality (e.g., Gagnon and Simon, 1974). But the long-term trend to assimilate the study of human sexuality to natural science and medicine, and to treat sexuality as a bundle of discrete 'behaviours', has had a powerful influence on AIDS research in the social sciences. It has been common in survey studies for sexuality to be measured by one, or at best a few, discrete items reporting particular behaviours — with little consideration of the interpersonal and cultural meanings of these actions, their character as social transactions, or their larger social contexts.

At the time we designed our questionnaire and carried out our interviews, little was known about the practice of sex among gay/

bisexual men. We would argue that a rational policy for the prevention of HIV infection must be informed by accurate information about such practice, including its meaning, patterning and social context. Human sexuality does not consist of separate, isolated items of behaviour. In real life a person's sexuality involves a complex of actions, emotions and relationships. Particular practices (such as unprotected anal intercourse) *always* occur in a wider repertoire of sexual and social activities. To change that particular practice requires a reshaping of the wider pattern of sexuality. This has not often been acknowledged or investigated in HIV/AIDS research. A major goal of the SAPA project, therefore, was to draw a map of the wider realm of sexuality, including the points of danger, as a guide for prevention workers.

The rise of a 'social constructionist' view of sexuality in the last two decades has been important in offering an alternative to positivist sexology. As we have argued in more detail in a theoretical essay (Connell and Dowsett, 1992), it is crucial not to represent sexuality through the logical couple 'social frame'/'biological basis'. Rather, we must see sexual activity as inherently social practice, a kind of practice through which living bodies are incorporated into social relations. In such an approach we become concerned with the politics of the transactions between embodied persons. Our argument on this theme will emphasize the issue of reciprocity in gay sexuality as a possible basis for a response to the epidemic which is consciously democratic.

In making this analysis we wish to emphasize the variety of possible types of sexuality. Cross-cultural research has dramatized the range of human sexualities, as seen in the notable work on homosexuality in Melanesia by Herdt (1981) and in the United States by W.L. Williams (1986). Within Western European culture, sex research has also been fertile in ideas about different styles of sexuality. Psychoanalysis has traditionally distinguished oral, anal and genital stages of sexual development and proposed that adult sexuality might become organized around (or fixated on) any of these foci or zones. A hierarchy of practices (in terms of pleasure or involvement) may emerge from what Freud (1964b) wryly called the 'polymorphously perverse disposition' of the child. Marcuse (1955) made the important theoretical suggestion that this emergence is socially structured. He hypothesized that the 'performance principle' in industrial civilization narrowly channels sexuality towards reproductive ends, gives a primacy to genital activity, and represses other aspects of sexuality as 'perversion'.

Erikson (1965) urged that Freudian concepts such as *orality* also refer to styles or modalities of interaction. One distinction of modality or mode has been very important in some conceptions of male homosexuality, that between 'passive' and 'active'. While this distinction has been greatly exaggerated as a guide to homosexual relationships, an 'insertive'/'receptive' distinction is also made within Western culture between mainstream and stigmatized sexual practices — though the boundaries shift over time, as Rubin's (1976) evidence on oral sex indicates. Here the emergence of *sexual subcultures* is at issue, a theme emphasized by Weeks (1986). We shall explore in our data statistical indications of these kinds of variations in sexuality as they apply to gay/bisexual men.

The Inventory of Sexual Practices

The study's major source of information on sexual conduct was an inventory of items on sexual practices, which was explored in the interview from several points of view. As a result of the pilot interviews, we adapted from Campbell *et al.* (1986) the device of using the layout of the questionnaire to distinguish general categories of practice from details subsumed under them. For instance, the section of the inventory on unprotected anal intercourse looked like this:

03. Anal Intercourse (Fucking) without condoms

      1. Active-giving (fucking partner and coming inside)
      2. Receiving (being fucked with partner coming)

The inventory contained sixteen general categories of practice, with forty specific categories, making fifty-six items in all, which are listed in Table 5.1. In the course of the interview, the interviewer worked through the full inventory up to seven times, with different orienting questions. The three which are of most concern here were specified as being about *sex with men* in one's private sex life:

1 *Experience/enjoyment*: 'With each one, could you tell me if you have tried it — and if you have, how much you enjoyed it?' (three-point rating scale)
2 *Frequency: regular partner*: 'How often in the last six months have you done any of the activities below with your regular male partners?' (three-point rating scale)

3   *Frequency: casual partner*: 'How often in the last six months have you done any of the activities below with your casual male partners?' (three-point rating scale)

The other 'runs' with the full inventory (modified where neces-sary in sections on sex with women) concerned *safety of sexual practices with men, experience/enjoyment with women, safety with women* and *sex with prostitutes*.

A shorter form of the inventory was used in a section asking about changes in practice made in response to awareness of AIDS. The general items of the full inventory were used as the basis for appraisal questions about the most satisfying practices. Those of relevance here are:

4   (*with men*) 'Of all the sexual activities you enjoy, which two do you find the most physically satisfying?'
5   (*with men*) 'Of all the sexual activities you enjoy, which two do you find the most emotionally satisfying?'

Besides the inventory, specific questions were asked about a number of aspects of sexual practice: anal and vaginal intercourse, frequency of sex, number of partners, communication during sexual encounters, early sexual experience, sex with women, prostitution, drug use when having sex, and sexually transmitted disease experience and precau-tions. All told, the questionnaire included 505 items concerned with aspects of sexual practice.

The Repertoire

An outline of the sexual experience of the men in the sample is pro-vided by Table 5.1, column A. Practices (general categories) are listed in order of the percentage who reported that they had ever tried them. This simple frequency count reveals three groups of practices: (i) those which were part of universal or almost universal *experience* in the sample, ranging from kissing and oral-genital sex to mutual masturba-tion and unprotected anal intercourse; (ii) a range of activities that were part of the majority *experience* without being universal, from rimming, through anal intercourse without ejaculation, to the use of sex toys; (iii) sexual activities that were part of the *experience* only of a small minority: SM/bondage, scat and watersports.

There was a difference between what people had experienced

Table 5.1. The Sexual Repertoire

Percentage who had engaged in each practice in sex with men. All items are general categories from the inventory of sexual practices apart from those marked 's' for specific category (n = 535)

	A Ever	B	C	D
			In past six months	
		With regular partner	With casual partner	With either regular or casual partner
Kissing	100	55	68	92
Oral-genital sex	100	53	69	92
Masturbation by self	100	(n.a.)	(n.a.)	(n.a.)
Sensuous touching	100	55	72	94
Mutual masturbation	98	53	67	90
Anal intercourse without condoms	95	31	24	48
Fantasy (e.g. pornography)	95	37	45	67
Oral-anal contact	86	25	22	40
Anal intercourse with condoms	81	28	44	59
Fingering the rectum[s]	80	32	34	54
Anal intercourse without coming	79	25	26	43
Sex aids	53	12	9	18
Cock-ring[s]	51	17	15	25
SM/bondage without blood	36	11	8	15
Fisting the rectum[s]	35	5	8	11
Watersports	29	5	2	7
SM/bondage with blood	12	1	1	2
Scat (sex with faeces)	7	1	1	2

Source: Connell and Kippax (1990).

and what they currently did. Though 86 per cent of the sample had experienced oral-anal contact, 20 per cent said they did not like it in the insertive mode, and 13 per cent said they did not like it in the receptive mode. Other circumstances such as the availability of partners and the impact of the HIV epidemic itself affected what was in the current repertoire. So a lower proportion, in this instance 40 per cent, had oral-anal contact as part of their current sexual repertoire compared with the 86 per cent who had tried it at some time.

Columns B, C and D in Table 5.1 show the range of sexual practices reported over the six months before the interview. To produce column D (the current repertoire), composite variables were constructed for each major category. In all cases the frequencies were lower than in column A.

The most common practices in the current repertoire were kissing, sensuous touching, masturbation and oral-genital sex. These four practices were engaged in by over 90 per cent of the men in the sample. Anal intercourse in all its forms, e.g., oral-anal contact, fingering the rectum and fantasy (which commonly includes anal-oriented pornography), was next in line, and in each case approximately half the men included the practice in their current repertoire. The remaining sexual practices, such as fisting the rectum, scat and watersports, were not at all popular.

Changes in the relative position of items within each column are of particular interest. Most notably, anal intercourse without condoms was sharply down in relative frequency. Compare, for instance, its numerical relationship to mutual masturbation in column A and in columns B, C and D. It is likely that this reflects the reception of the 'safe sex' message, documented in other parts of this study. Indeed, with the exceptions of kissing, oral-genital sex, sensuous touching and masturbation, all sexual practices had a markedly lower frequency in columns B, C and D than in column A. The average current repertoire was distinctly lower than total experience.

It is clear from columns B and C of Table 5.1 that the repertoire with 'regular' and with 'casual' partners was very similar. In general, it was not the case that respondents sought one kind of partner for one practice and another kind of partner for another. The major difference between the two lists was in the indications of greater caution with casual partners, particularly in relation to anal intercourse (less unprotected, more protected). The lower frequencies with casual partners for rimming, SM/bondage and watersports might also be interpreted in this way. With regard to these esoteric or minority practices, an equally plausible interpretation is that men who enjoy these activities found it relatively difficult to find like-interested partners. They had more opportunity to engage in these practices if they had a regular partner with similar sexual interests.

Is there any evidence that men who were losing desired outlets were turning to prostitutes for them? Only 6 per cent of respondents reported having paid for sex in the previous year, but it is still possible to explore relative frequencies. There is no evidence for a 'displacement of unsafe sex' hypothesis. The numbers were small, and the practices which reached even a 1 per cent level of demand were those which were a universal part of sexual experience generally: kissing, oral-genital sex, etc. On this evidence one would not be especially concerned about prostitution as a pathway of HIV transmission in the population tapped by this sample. Whether the same is true for other populations is another matter.

Table 5.2. Enjoyment

Percentage who rated each practice *very enjoyable* and *not enjoyable* (top and bottom categories in three-point scale) (n = 535)

	Very enjoyable	Not enjoyable
Kissing	76	1
Oral-genital sex	79	2
Masturbation by self	51	6
Sensuous touching	90	1
Mutual masturbation	60	3
Anal intercourse without condom	70	6
Fantasy	41	6
Oral-anal contact	40	14
Anal intercourse with condom	28	15
Anal intercourse without coming	25	17
Fisting or fingering the rectum	24	14
Using sex aids/cock rings	18	16
SM/bondage without blood	9	10
Watersports	4	13
SM/bondage with blood	2	8
Scat	0	7

Source: Connell and Kippax (1990).

The Emotional Profile of Sexuality

What people *do* sexually is not necessarily what they most enjoy or most value. Accordingly, we asked further questions about the emotional meanings of the practices in the repertoire. In the first place we asked respondents to rate each activity in terms of pleasure, on a three-point scale. Table 5.2 presents, for major categories, the percentages who rated each practice as *very enjoyable* and the percentage who rated it *not enjoyable*. The items are presented in order of frequency *ever done* as shown in Table 5.1.

Only one practice approached universal endorsement as highly pleasurable: sensuous touching. (The specific category that approached this level is *massage, caressing, cuddling*.) This fact points to the *relational* character of sex for the men interviewed. This response would not be expected if their sexuality were mainly organized around 'impersonal' sex. Also significant on this count was the high rating for kissing.

Oral-genital sex and anal intercourse *without* condoms ranked reasonably high for enjoyment. In contrast, anal intercourse *with* condoms was rated as very enjoyable by only 28 per cent of the sample. In fact, 15 per cent rated anal intercourse *with* condoms *not enjoyable*, a relatively high frequency of rejection.

Table 5.3.   Satisfaction

Percentage who cited each practice as one of the two *most physically satisfying* or one of the two most *emotionally satisfying* (n = 535)

	Most physically satisfying	Most emotionally satisfying
Kissing	14	37
Oral-genital sex	49	23
Masturbation by self	7	3
Sensuous touching	27	59
Mutual masturbation	16	10
Anal intercourse without condom	54	36
Fantasy	2	3
Oral-anal contact	6	3
Anal intercourse with condom	11	8
Anal intercourse without coming	3	1
Fisting or fingering the rectum	3	1
Using sex aids/cock rings	1	1
SM/bondage without blood	2	2
Watersports	0	0
SM/bondage with blood	0	0
Scat	0	0

Source: Connell and Kippax (1990).

The overall pattern of these ratings implies a capacity for gaining pleasure from a broad spectrum of activities. This is promising from the viewpoint of AIDS prevention strategies that seek to replace high-risk practices with low-risk ones.

To investigate whether there were particular foci of emotion among these practices, we next asked respondents to look over the whole inventory and identify the two sexual practices *most physically* and the two *most emotionally satisfying*. The tally of *most physically satisfying* responses is shown in the first column of Table 5.3. The two practices that stood out far above the rest were anal intercourse and oral-genital sex; both commonly lead to orgasm. This pattern is very different from the pattern of genital primacy identified by Marcuse (1955), whose argument treated homoeroticism as part of what was socially repressed. It is striking to find so marked a pattern in a sample of gay and bisexual men. Our finding raises the possibility of some convergence between the sexual expression of gay and 'straight' masculinities over the last generation, in the context of the social reconstitution of homosexuality traced by Altman (1979, 1982). Both practices necessitate an insertive and a receptive partner.

The dilemmas of 'safe sex' HIV prevention strategies are dramatically shown in these figures. One of the practices (anal intercourse without condoms) which had the highest proportion of gay and bisexual men rating it as *most physically satisfying* is also the most dangerous. The obvious replacement, anal intercourse with condoms, was nominated as most physically satisfying by only one in ten of the sample. The other practice, oral-genital sex, which was an erotic focus for a comparable number, is of uncertain safety. Both practices involve ejaculation and the exchange of body fluids.

Sexual exotica were a focus for a small minority. Fantasy sex (the general category includes pornography, as well as dressing up) does not appear a credible line of development for safe sex strategy — there was an enormous difference between the numbers who had tried it (Table 5.1) and those who found it enjoyable or most satisfying (Tables 5.2 and 5.3). Perhaps the most consoling figures here are those that showed that other practices with a degree of risk — fisting, anal intercourse without ejaculation, SM/bondage with blood — had not established themselves as erotic foci for many in the sample. As we show in Chapter 11, these practices have dropped in frequency when compared with five years before. There is also something positive in the fact that two safe practices — mutual masturbation and sensuous touching — were next in line as foci after anal intercourse and oral-genital sex, though at only half the frequency.

Judgments of *most emotionally satisfying* are tallied in the second column of Table 5.3. The most common emotional focus by far was sensuous touching. Next came kissing, then anal intercourse without condoms; further back, oral-genital sex; the rest comparatively nowhere. Some practices on which hope had been placed as a 'safe sex' displacement, such as mutual masturbation and protected anal intercourse, were emotional foci only for one in ten respondents — not a large base to build from.

It would appear that in terms of emotional satisfaction the primacy of anal and oral-genital sex has been overlaid by, and to some extent displaced by, a pattern of *communicative primacy*. In sensuous touching and in kissing, the sense of whole persons in contact, not just bodies, is particularly strong. The other practice in the inventory with strong communicative character (fantasy) stresses the imaginary rather than the real personal contact and ranked low on emotional satisfaction. The form of safe sex which is *least* communicative (solo masturbation) ranked low as a focus of emotional satisfaction. The possibility that the communicative dimension of sexuality might be a major source of positive sexual pleasure, if it can be sustained, has important implications for HIV/AIDS prevention work which seeks to present a pro-sex message.

Types of Sexuality Based on Experience/Enjoyment

We have mentioned three theoretical types of patterning in sexuality, by *erotic zone*, by *mode* and by *social definition*. A study of the inter-correlation of items in the inventory casts light on the presence or absence of these patterns. Respondents were asked to rate their enjoyment of each sexual activity on a three-point scale. In this analysis, *no experience* was included with the lowest level of enjoyment. The variable of experience/enjoyment is presumed to define the level of pleasurable involvement in a particular practice. A forty-six by forty-six correlation matrix, based on the specific practice items in the inventory, was calculated.

Mode

If mode were the major pattern of differentiation in gay sexuality, then correlations between one insertive practice and other insertive practices should be higher than the correlation between that practice and its matched receptive practice. If, on the contrary, the correlations between matched insertive and receptive practices were higher than correlations among insertive (or among receptive) practices, we would conclude that other forms of differentiation are stronger. Such a pattern might suggest the importance of a practice or ethic of reciprocity within gay relationships, where partners exchange modes in relation to the same practices.

The highest correlations were almost without exception between different specific categories under the same general category, or between variations on the same physical performance. A section of the matrix dealing with oral-genital sex and anal intercourse is shown in Appendix 4A, where this pattern can be seen. Generally, the strongest relationships were between receptive and insertive modes of the same practices. This pattern was very general in the larger matrix and suggests that pleasurable involvement is organized around types of practice more than around mode of that practice. Thus, for instance, the correlation of insertive oral-genital contact with receptive oral-genital contact was much stronger than the correlation between insertive oral-genital contact and insertive anal intercourse. Indeed, the strongest associations between oral-genital sex and anal intercourse were between those practices which involve ejaculation and those which do not. It was clear that the mode effect was at best weak.

There was, nevertheless, some suggestion of a mode effect; but the modal pattern occurs only *within* a set of practices, with the same or similar physical performance. For the anal intercourse items in Appendix 4A, the coefficients between items of the same mode were noticeably higher than those between items of opposite mode, and on a par with those between the insertive and receptive modes for each practice. The oral-genital items did not follow the modal pattern. This analysis suggests that we should think of a mode as specific to the enjoyment of anal intercourse and not as a general feature of sexuality or personality.

Social Definition

In the overall inter-item correlation matrix, only one well defined grouping of items emerged: watersports, SM/bondage and fisting the rectum, with firm links to scat and use of dildos. A pattern of adventurous or 'heavy' sex was suggested. Few of the men in our sample had ever experienced these activities (see Table 5.1); hence we call them 'esoteric' sexual practices. The item intercorrelations reflected the presence of a large number of men who had never experienced these activities and a small minority who had experienced several. The picture suggested a subcultural organization of sexuality.

Erotic Zone

No other cluster of items was very strong. A factor analysis of the enjoyment/experience items yielded a strong factor of esoteric sexual practices, but no others that would produce robust scales.

Two interesting patterns thus emerged from the data on pleasurable involvement. First, mode was not important except in relation to anal intercourse. Instead, reciprocity was important in structuring sexual pleasure. Second, there appeared to be a subcultural pattern of enjoyment of esoteric practice. Apart from these, no broad patterns of differentiation were shown. Men in the sample gained pleasure from a wide spectrum of sexual practices. These data do not point to early cathexes which fix later experience, as in much psychoanalytic thinking about sexuality. Rather, pleasurable involvement embraces the three erotic zones: anal, oral and genital.

Types of Sexuality Based on Current Practice

The analysis of the repertoire and the emotional profile indicated an important distinction between the extent to which a particular practice occurred and the emotional investment in it. Accordingly, we conducted a separate investigation of types of sexuality through analysis of the inventory items scored in terms of current practice. The organization of practices on this basis proved more clearcut than the organization of pleasure just discussed.

Questions about frequency of practices had been asked separately in relation to regular and casual partners, and not everybody in the sample had both. Further, the classification of respondents on the basis of relationship status was based on a question about current relationships, but the frequency questions in the inventory of sexual practices asked about practice *in the last six months*, resulting in some people (correctly) answering frequency questions about a relationship which no longer existed. Clearly, it was desirable to amalgamate the questions if possible. Separate factor analyses were conducted on the two subpopulations answering questions about casual and regular partners, and factor structures were found that were so similar that we had no hesitation in collapsing the data and treating all the questions as defining a single sexual repertoire. Since we were examining how many *different* activities were engaged in, we did not consider it appropriate to regard anal intercourse with a condom and without a condom as constituting *two* practices. The issue of condom use (or non-use) is addressed in the section on 'danger' in Chapter 6.

Three groups of items emerged from our analysis of *practices*: a group of *tactile and oral* sexual practices (kissing, oral-genital sex, mutual masturbation, sensuous touching); a group of *anal* practices (oral-anal contact, fingering the rectum, anal intercourse); and a group of relatively rare *esoteric* practices (watersports, fisting the rectum, SM/ bondage). These groupings were sufficiently well defined to allow the construction of scales, a great convenience in our analysis and in using this study as a baseline in further research. The *casual* and *regular* items were amalgamated to produce three composite scales, which we call Oral/Tactile Practices (OTP), Essentially Anal Practices (EAP) and Infrequent Esoteric Practices (IEP).

Characteristics of the scales are shown in Table 5.4, and details of the scoring of the items may be found in Appendix 5. Scale scores represent the *extent* of sexual activity within the particular type defined by the scale. (A person who was celibate for the last six months should score zero on each scale.) Distributions of scores on the oral/tactile

Table 5.4. Details of Sexual Practice Scales

	Item mean	Item-total correlation
Oral/Tactile Practices (OTP)		
1 Wet kissing/deep kissing	0.89	.67
2 Dry kissing	0.86	.54
3 Sucking (oral-genital)*	0.87	.68
4 Being sucked (oral-genital)*	0.88	.64
5 Masturbating (jerking off) together	0.90	.61
6 Sensuous touching	0.94	.79
* Either with or without ejaculation		
Essentially Anal Practices (EAP)		
1 Oral-anal contact (rimming/roseleafing your partner) (giving)	0.31	.47
2 Oral-anal contact (being rimmed/roseleafed) (receiving)	0.36	.46
3 Anal intercourse (fucking): active-giving (fucking partner and coming inside)*	0.66	.49
4 Anal intercourse (fucking): receiving (being fucked with partner coming)	0.62	.50
5 Anal intercourse (fucking): without ejaculation (coming): active-giving (fucking partner without coming inside)	0.38	.51
6 Anal intercourse (fucking): without ejaculation (coming): receiving (being fucked without partner coming)	0.34	.47
7 Finger in partner's rectum (finger fucking)	0.51	.54
8 Finger in your rectum (being finger fucked)	0.49	.55
* Either with or without condom		
Infrequent Esoteric Practices (IEP)		
1 Having your partner urinate on you (watersports)	0.05	.53
2 Urinating on your partner	0.05	.50
3 Fisting partner (hand/fist in partner's rectum)	0.10	.42
4 Being fisted (hand/fist in your rectum)	0.05	.44
5 Receiving dildo/vibrator/toy	0.15	.63
6 Giving dildo/vibrator/toy	0.15	.63
7 S/M dominance/bondage: giving (top)*	0.12	.56
8 S/M dominance/bondage: receiving (bottom)*	0.13	.57
* Either with or without blood		

Scale characteristics

	Number of items	Range possible	Mean score	Standard deviation	Alpha
Oral/Tactile Practices (OTP)	6	0–6	5.3	1.4	0.86
Essentially Anal Practices (EAP)	8	0–6	3.7	2.5	0.79
Infrequent Esoteric Practices (IEP)	8	0–8	0.8	1.5	0.81

Intercorrelations	OTP	EAP	IEP
OTP	1.00	0.44	0.15
EAP		1.00	0.42
IEP			1.00

Source: Connell and Kippax (1990).

(OTP) and esoteric practice (IEP) scales were skewed, reflecting the high numbers of people who engaged in the former and low numbers who engaged in the latter. Nevertheless, the three scales all achieved satisfactory reliability.

The Oral/Tactile Practices (OTP) scale appeared the most complex. It includes items relating to oral sex (kissing and oral-genital sex), but it also incudes mutual masturbation and sensuous touching. One of its items, oral-genital sex, was shown above (Table 5.3) to be one of the most physically satisfying practices, while another two, sensuous touching and kissing, were the two most emotionally satisfying practices. One might see this scale as particularly connected with the interpersonal dimension of sex. None of the practices is socially forbidden, except in the sense that gay sex as such is. Within Australian gay communities these practices are not subject to censure and are acceptable to all. At the same time, these items might be characterized as a 'safe sex' cluster. The scale contains the items which were almost universally practised. The correlation of this scale with the EAP scale was reasonably high, but it had only a small correlation with the IEP scale.

The Essentially Anal Practices (EAP) scale was easier to interpret and label. It contains nearly all the items focused on anal practices: oral-anal contact, fingering the rectum and all the anal intercourse items. It does not, however, include the use of sex toys or dildos, or fisting. It contains one of the practices which many found both physically and emotionally satisfying, namely anal intercourse. The items included in this scale were not practised universally, but they were each practised by at least half the men in the sample.

The Infrequent Esoteric Practices (IEP) scale contains almost all the esoteric practices which emerged in our analysis of pleasurable involvement, with the exception of scat. This scale can be interpreted as measuring engagement in a rather specific subcultural world. It is clear that, in this instance, the organization of pleasure and practice are almost identical. The scale had a very low mean (see Table 5.4); very few men engaged in these activities.

The analysis pointed to two major patterns in relation to frequency of sexual practice, which are the basis of scales OTP and EAP. It is tempting to see this as reflecting differences in zonal orientation, calling the one scale 'oral' and the other 'anal'. However, there is more to it than that. The first scale is an oral *and* tactile sex scale. It includes practices which satisfy both emotional and physical desire and, as well, may reflect the availability of partners. It contains the relatively safe practices, and almost all of the men in the sample engaged in *most* of them. The second scale seems focused on anal intercourse and has a more obvious zonal interpretation. Even here, however, more than zone is at issue. This scale contains the most risky of the practices. As the scale means indicated, markedly fewer men in the sample engaged in those practices to any great degree. It is possible that doing a lot of different things in the area of oral-tactile practice and fewer in the anal-erotic area represents a reorganization of sexual practice in response to the HIV epidemic.

As well as the existence of these scales, and in part responsible for their existence, was the finding from the pattern of correlation coefficients between practices that reciprocity was an even more important organizing construct in practice than it was in pleasure. The strongest correlations were between insertive and receptive modes of each practice, and the modal pattern of correlation was noticeably absent.

Relationship between Pleasure and Practice

Our analysis has presented two aspects of sexuality: one that deals with pleasure and the other with practice. Sexual *practice*, in a very general sense, appeared focused on oral and tactile sex, these practices being almost universal, as well as on anal sex. There was also a small group of men who engaged in esoteric practices. A second pattern was associated with *pleasure*: physical pleasure, which was focused on anal intercourse and oral-genital sex; and emotional pleasure, which was focused on communicative primacy, and included sensuous touching, kissing and anal intercourse.

With the exception of those who engaged in esoteric sex, men in our sample did not always do the things they liked, nor always enjoy the things that they did. It seemed important to make a systematic analysis of the link between pleasure and practice. Accordingly, we listed practices in order of enjoyment, and then calculated the percentages, of those who said they enjoyed a practice, who actually engaged in it. The results of this calculation are shown in Table 5.5.

The item-by-item analysis shows that:

1 'safe' sex (defined in terms of AIDS educators' knowledge at the time of the survey) — kissing, anal intercourse with condoms, oral-genital sex without ejaculation, mutual masturbation, sensuous touching and fingering the rectum — was practised by 70–95 per cent of those who enjoyed it;

Table 5.5. *Enjoyment by Sexual Practice* (n = 535)

Sexual practice	Of total sample, percentage who report practice very enjoyable or quite enjoyable	Of those who enjoy, percentage who actually engage in practice (often or occasionally)
Sensuous touching	98.7	94.5
Dry kissing	83.5	91.1
Wet kissing	95.5	90.8
Mutual masturbation	95.5	91.8
Oral-genital (insertive no ejaculation)	92.0	87.4
Oral-genital (receptive no semen)	92.2	85.4
Oral-genital (insertive with ejaculation)	85.4	45.1
Oral-genital (receptive with semen)	56.2	47.2
Fingering the rectum (insertive)	65.0	71.0
Fingering the rectum (receptive)	61.7	69.4
Anal intercourse (insertive with condoms)	58.7	72.9
Anal intercourse (receptive with condoms)	52.8	72.8
Anal intercourse (insertive no condoms)	84.0	44.3
Anal intercourse (receptive no condoms)	72.9	42.3
Anal intercourse (insertive no ejaculation)	54.8	52.6
Anal intercourse (receptive no semen)	51.6	52.2
Oral-anal (insertive)	57.2	48.0
Oral-anal (receptive)	72.7	43.7
Use of toys (insertive)	30.3	43.2
Use of toys (receptive)	31.6	30.2
Fisting (insertive)	22.2	35.3
Fisting (receptive)	8.9	39.6
SM/bondage with blood (top)	22.8	44.3
SM/bondage with blood (bottom)	23.2	49.2
Watersports (giving)	14.6	29.5
Watersports (receptive)	12.9	31.9

Source: Connell and Kippax (1990).

2 'unsafe' sex — anal intercourse without ejaculation, anal intercourse without condoms, oral-genital with ejaculation, toys, SM/bondage with blood and fisting — was practised by 35–55 per cent of those who enjoyed it. For example, 84 per cent of the sample said they enjoyed insertive anal intercourse without condoms, but only 44 per cent of those who enjoyed it engaged in this activity; and

3 esoteric sex, such as watersports, was practised by only 20 per cent of those who said they enjoyed it. Perhaps there is a difficulty of finding partners, as well as an assumption of danger.

These figures also pointed to a distinction which respondents drew with regard to the enjoyment of the insertive and receptive mode of three 'unsafe' sexual practices. Insertive oral-genital sex with ejaculation was enjoyed by many more men than its more unsafe receptive

counterpart. Similarly, insertive fisting was enjoyed by more men than receptive fisting. Receptive oral-anal contact was enjoyed by more men than receptive fisting; receptive oral-anal contact was enjoyed by more men than insertive oral-anal contact. These three practices were the only three to show this difference. Although at first glance the distinction is related to risk (from hepatitis as well as HIV), such as explanation is not the whole story. If it were, we should expect to find a distinction between insertive and receptive modes of anal intercourse, for example. Many men did not find either the insertive mode of oral-anal contact or the receptive mode of fisting and oral-genital sex enjoyable.

Whatever the explanation of the above insertive/receptive distinctions, two things are clear. Sexual practice for gay men involves reciprocation. The majority of men enjoyed all their sexual activities, but in those cases where there was a preference, men practised both the insertive and receptive modes, even if they did not enjoy both.

Further, the more general analysis of the relationship between practice and enjoyment made it clear that many men had changed their sexual practices. As we show in Chapters 6 and 7, they had given up or modified those unsafe practices which they enjoy. Practice has been modified by a rational fear of HIV transmission.

Conclusions and Implications for AIDS Prevention

The patterns of sexuality traced in this chapter go some way towards explaining the shape of the AIDS crisis among gay men. The significance of anal intercourse in both physical and emotional enjoyment places the most risky sexual practice close to the heart of the social process of constructing gayness. The evidence shows the emotional charge still attached to anal practices. As we show later, though difficult, it is possible to change sexual practices.

Our findings in this chapter suggest some constructive lines of development for preventive work. There are different sources of pleasure within sexuality. Preventive work might seek to build on the inherent gratifications of oral sex (without ejaculation), a form of genital sex which is generally considered safe. The emotional satisfaction derived from communicative sex deserves attention. It is notable that sensuous touching, the practice that ranks highest for *emotionally satisfying*, is also the practice that received near-universal endorsement as *very enjoyable*.

We are not suggesting that there is a separate group of communicative practices which can be substituted for others. Rather, we are suggesting that the communicative dimension inherent in *all* sexual practices be emphasized as a source of pleasure. Besides confirming current practice and eroticizing condoms, one might emphasize the communicative aspect of anal sex as not necessarily being affected by condom use. Such an approach would build on a notable feature of the HIV epidemic so far, the strength of gay men's collective response to it.

Sexuality is, notoriously, not a realm where cold rational judgments of self-interest hold sway. This point has often been made by stressing the irrationality of lust and love, their connections with unconscious motivation or biological impulse. In the perspective developed in this chapter, the point is rather that sexuality is the bearer of a very complex and contradictory set of socially constructed emotions and attachments. An overrationalistic 'safe sex' policy in effect wishes away this reality. The point is rather to reshape it, to use the social dimension of sexuality to build *sustainable* safe sex regimes, as we argue at more length in Chapter 11.

This becomes a practical proposition to the extent that other kinds of gratification can be found. The importance of anal sex can be exaggerated. The gay/bisexual repertoire is much wider, and has other foci as well. Here the findings about sexuality, especially the potential importance of communicative eroticism, converge with the findings on information and gay community connections. A feasible prevention strategy might be centred on the relational dimension of sexuality, and the need for informed social support for social practice — where knowledge about HIV/AIDS issues comes via (or is discussed in) relationships that also provide encouragement and personal back-up for changed practice.

We need to move beyond the individualist emphasis of much official health education and academic AIDS research, towards collective, social strategies of change. The aim of such work is not so much to change individual 'attitudes' or 'health behaviours' as to move whole networks of people towards safe practice, and to encourage the social processes among them which can sustain the prevention.

There are many indications in our data of the vigour of responses to the AIDS crisis. The relationship between enjoyment and practice (Table 5.5) points to the active response of gay men. The pattern of reciprocity in gay sexuality holds promise for modification of practice; negotiation is likely to be easier in relationships where there is reciprocal sexual practice. This, along with the social networks constructing

gay communities, may be seen as the base for the powerful collective response that has been made to the epidemic — a response which must continue, as our data on unsafe practice, discussed in the next chapter, will confirm.

Chapter 6

Correlates of Sexual Practice:
Safe and Unsafe

The patterns of sexual pleasure and practice which we identified in the previous chapter raise questions about their generality. For example, if there are men who engage in very little (or very few practices involving) anal sex, are they distinguished from other men on the basis of structural variables, such as age, education, income, or on the basis of social setting, such as relationship status, place of residence? What variables (if any) distinguish those men who engage in infrequent esoteric practices from the remainder of the sample? Are there certain characteristics which differ between men who never practise unprotected anal intercourse and those who sometimes do so? Can we contribute to an understanding of the contexts in which unsafe sexual practice occurs? These are some of the questions which we explore in this chapter, together with a consideration of the implications for HIV/AIDS prevention arising out of our findings.

Social and Situational Correlates of Sexual Practice

A strategic question for AIDS prevention is how sexual practices vary between groups. If unsafe practice, for instance, is relatively concentrated in a particular social setting, a 'targeting' strategy would be suggested. A study of the social correlates of sexual practice may also suggest circumstances that lead to safe and unsafe practice. In examining these issues we cannot treat the social setting as fixed and unchanging. It is abundantly obvious that the gay community has itself been reshaped around the epidemic. Accordingly, we include alongside social structure variables and social milieu variables a number of items and scales that bear on the situation created by the epidemic itself.

The statistical relationships between these three sets of variables and the three scales of sexual practice are shown in Appendix 4B. We will consider first the IEP (Infrequent Esoteric Practices) and EAP (Essentially Anal Practices) scales. The small number of men who engaged in the esoteric practices can be characterized on some structure variables. They tended to be middle-aged men who were Australian or of English-speaking background and of Protestant religious persuasion. Although the pattern of differences on the anal practice scale paralleled that on the esoteric scale, the differences were not significant. Men with high rather than a very low income, however, were more likely to have a high score on the anal scale.

When we turn to the contextual and situational variables, there is a sense in which men who engaged most in the anal practices, and those who engaged in the esoteric practices, fit the stereotype of the 'fast lane' gay man. Men who had a large number of gay male friends, who had more personal contact with the epidemic and had been tested were likely to have engaged in a wider variety of esoteric and anal practices. Further, they seemed to be more closely tied to the Oxford Street community (although not a statistically significant result) and were more likely to recognize AIDS pamphlets. Those men who rated anal sex as very important to them were also likely to have engaged in more esoteric sexual practices.

So in one sense the stereotype of the 'fast lane' gay man was confirmed. However, in two extremely important ways it is an inaccurate picture of contemporary gay sexuality. First, both esoteric and anal practices were more common within regular and monogamous relationships; men who had only casual sex engaged in these practices to a lesser extent. Second, only half the men in the sample engaged in anal practices and extremely few men practised esoteric sex. It is the oral/tactile practices which most accurately characterized the sexual practice of the majority of gay men in our sample.

With regard to the oral/tactile practices, few among the structural variables distinguished those who practised these activities from those who did not. High scores had a consistent but non-significant association with income and a significant association with education. Among situational variables, OTP was linked with the general issues (GI) scale, which measures caution (as opposed to rashness or optimism) with regard to opinions about the HIV epidemic. As one might expect, men who scored high on the OTP scale were more likely than others to be cautious. The clearest links with oral/tactile practices were among the milieu variables, where high scores were associated with high sexual and social engagement in gay community.

A positive relationship was found between education and income on the one hand and variety of sexual practice on the other. As well, there were significant relationships between number of gay male friends and all the practice scales. These results indicated that men who were economically and socially secure had a wider and more varied sexual practice than men who were not so secure.

In summary, structural variables appeared to have little impact on the sexual practices of our sample. There were more links between the practice scales and the milieu variables. These mainly concern the variables that directly describe the social organization of sexuality or sexual relationships. It is not surprising, in a general sense, to find practice embedded in relationship. What is interesting here are the indications of the specific kinds of relatedness that give rise to high levels of sexual activity: the presence of a 'relationship' and friendship base (perhaps, again, providing security) is important.

Correlates of Sexual Pleasure

The measures of enjoyment or pleasure produced a slightly different picture from the frequency of practice measures. As respondents were asked to nominate the two most physically and emotionally satisfying practices, the categories of practice were collapsed in terms of the empirically most frequent pairings. The three sets of contextual variables — structure, milieu and situation — were cross-classified with those practices in the inventory chosen for physical satisfaction, and separately for emotional satisfaction. Emotional pleasure and physical pleasure were closely related: those who find a practice emotionally satisfying were highly likely to find that same practice physically satisfying. The one exception was kissing and sensuous touching. Those who endorsed these practices as one of the two most emotionally satisfying found a wide range of practices other than these physically satisfying. With one or two exceptions, the situation and milieu variables did not show significant associations. Importance of anal intercourse and antibody status were, as one might expect, significantly related to choosing anal intercourse without condoms as most physically and emotionally satisfying.

The major finding was that pleasure, particularly emotional pleasure, was associated with a number of structural variables. Age was significantly related to which practices were nominated as emotionally ($p < 0.0005$) and physically ($p < 0.03$) satisfying. Young (20–29) gay and bisexual men were less likely to nominate anal intercourse without condoms and more likely to nominate kissing and sensuous touching as the most emotionally and physically satisfying, while older men (40 plus) were more likely to nominate anal intercourse without condoms and less likely to nominate kissing and sensuous touching as the most satisfying.

Nomination of anal intercourse without condoms as emotionally satisfying was also significantly related to occupation ($p < 0.005$) and to education ($p < 0.006$). Men with least education and those in sales/ manual jobs were most likely to nominate anal intercourse without condoms and oral-genital sex as emotionally satisfying and least likely to nominate kissing and sensuous touching.

Clearly, enjoyment, particularly emotional enjoyment, is constituted within certain social contexts. Therefore, it can be reconstructed. Anal intercourse is structured differently for different men and over time. The data suggest that time has had an impact on the way in which sexual pleasure among these men is understood. Although they are difficult to unravel, there appear to be both a generational difference and a difference which is a function of maturity. Men who were sexually active during the so-called 'permissive' era find most sexual pleasure in anal intercourse without condoms, whereas younger men are more likely to find pleasure in sensuous touching and kissing. This latter finding may be due to lack of experience and, in that case, will change with time. It may also be a function of the impact of the HIV epidemic.

Dangerous Practice

It is generally recognized that anal intercourse without condoms has been the main means of transmission of HIV in male homosexual contexts. It is specifically identified in retrospective stories of cases of HIV infection as the main pathway of the epidemic in Australia. It is to anal intercourse without condoms, in particular, that we refer when we use the term 'dangerous'.

Some 95 per cent of our sample reported having experience of anal intercourse without condoms at some time in their lives. Much smaller, though still substantial, percentages reported having engaged in it 'within the last six months': 31 per cent with a regular sexual partner, 24 per cent with a casual partner. There is some overlap: 48 per cent had done it in this period with either regular or casual partner or both. Unprotected anal intercourse is thus more common among men in regular relationships. This seems broadly consistent with the finding from another Sydney cohort of gay men (Tindall *et al.*, 1989) that the

Table 6.1. Judgments of the Safety of Unprotected Anal Intercourse (n = 535)

	Practice is judged to be			
	Very safe	Small risk	Not at all safe	Unsure, don't know
	(percentages)			
Insertive with ejaculation	2	24	74	1
Receptive with ejaculation	1	5	94	0
Insertive without ejaculation	11	55	33	1
Receptive without ejaculation	9	49	42	1

Source: Connell *et al.* (1990)

tendency to have anal sex without condoms varies with type of partner, being more likely with partners presumed to be safe.

It was very widely known among our respondents that one modality of unprotected anal intercourse, in particular, was dangerous. Ninety-four per cent considered that *receptive* anal intercourse with ejaculation and without condoms was 'not at all safe', on a three-point rating scale. This was the highest 'unsafe' rating for any practice in a very detailed fifty-six-item inventory. It parallels findings in other studies, such as the Melbourne community survey reported by Sinnott and Todd (1988); this piece of information is widespread. Table 6.1 shows judgments of risk for this and three other closely related practices. Seventy-one per cent of respondents reported that they have started using condoms, or used condoms more, since becoming aware of AIDS — the highest rate of uptake of any new practice in a fourteen-item inventory on changes. Table 6.1 shows that judgments about the safety of the insertive partner were more sanguine for the receptive partner, and judgments of the safety of intercourse without ejaculating were markedly more sanguine.

How was dangerous practice related to the broader patterns of sexuality just described? To examine this, we cross-classified answers to a number of questions about frequency of unprotected anal intercourse with regular and casual partners, the importance of anal intercourse, and feelings about condoms. We also examined their connections with the three scales of sexual practice just described.

As it did not matter, with regard to HIV transmission, whether the respondent was the insertive or receptive partner or engaged in both activities, we constructed a composite variable distinguishing those who had any modality of unprotected anal intercourse (insertive or receptive) from those who did not. We called this variable 'danger in practice', and we examined this composite variable with respect to regular and casual partners. The results of this analysis are shown in Table 6.2. Most of the sexuality variables were linked to the danger measure. In the case of Essentially Anal Practices this occurs almost by definition, as anal intercourse is an item in that scale. The existence of the scale itself indicates a statistical connection of this practice to other 'anal' practices. What is perhaps more notable is that links were also found beyond this group.

Higher frequencies of sex with casual partners in the previous month were found in the 'high danger' group (presumably an 'opportunity' effect). The high danger group tended to think anal intercourse more important to them, and were less likely to find condoms acceptable. Perhaps most interesting was the relationship with infrequent esoteric practices (the IEP scale) in the case of casual partners, where the high danger group were more likely to be participants in this small sexual subculture. None of these relationships is counter-intuitive. Taken together, they point to the extent to which dangerous anal practice is embedded in a larger pattern of sexuality.

A separate analysis of structural correlates was conducted for the 'danger in practice' measure. The results are shown in detail in Appendix 4C. These variables had little connection with danger in anal practice. Only three relationships exceeded the .05 level of significance and one could be expected by chance alone. The age variable suggests a generational effect, but may reflect a greater willingness to have intercourse without condoms in long-established relationships. The finding for religion, with Protestant respondents more involved in unprotected intercourse with regular partners, is surprising. The occupation variable, together with non-significant trends in the same direction for education, indicated greater caution among the professionally trained. This is an interesting finding given that it was these same men who were more likely to engage in a wide variety of anal practice (see above). Broadly, the lack of connection between 'danger in practice' and structural variables argues against a 'targeting' strategy for prevention work, and in favour of broad-based programs – so far as subgroups within the population defined by this study are concerned.

Stronger statistical relationships were found with the variables describing interpersonal and social milieu. Relationship status, and all three variables relating to gay community (Sexual Engagement, Social Engagement and Community Involvement, to be described in detail in Chapter 9), were related to different patterns of unprotected anal sex. These findings point to several dynamics.

The first concerns 'monogamy' and is most clearly illustrated by the items on relationship status. Monogamy is indeed associated with

Table 6.2(a). Relationship of 'Danger in Anal Practice' to Other Aspects of Sexuality*

	Those with regular partners				Those with casual partners			
	High danger (either or both modes) %	Low danger (neither mode) %	n	p	High danger (either or both modes) %	Low danger (neither mode) %	n	p
How often had sex with casual partners in last month								
None/NR	58	42	65		20	80	150	
1–5 times	51	49	231		31	69	102	
6–15 times	47	53	78		37	63	36	
More than 15	40	60	20	ns	60	40	10	.005
Importance of anal intercourse in sex with men								
Very important	68	32	66		40	60	80	
Quite important	56	44	117		36	64	154	
Not important	46	54	88		28	72	121	
No response/don't know	33	67	27	.005	10	90	39	.005
Feeling about condoms in sex with men								
Completely acceptable	51	49	87		22	78	125	
Quite acceptable	56	44	171		35	65	216	
Quite or completely unacceptable	56	44	36	ns	48	52	46	.002

Table 6.2(b). Relationship of 'Danger in Anal Practice' to Other Aspects of Sexuality: Means and Standard Deviations

	Those with regular partners			Those with casual partners		
	High danger (either or both modes)	Low danger (neither mode)	p	High danger (either or both modes)	Low danger (neither mode)	p
	n = 160	n = 138		n = 125	n = 269	
Sexuality scales						
Essentially Anal Practice (EAP)						
Mean:	5.2	3.4	.0000	5.0	3.2	.0000
SD:	2.1	2.4		2.0	2.3	
Oral/Tactile Practice (OTP)						
Mean:	5.8	5.6	.07	5.7	5.6	ns
SD:	0.5	0.9		0.7	0.8	
Infrequent Esoteric Practice (IEP)						
Mean:	1.2	1.0	ns	1.0	0.7	.02
SD:	1.9	1.7		1.7	1.4	

Note: 'Danger' measure is whether the respondent had had unprotected anal intercourse (insertive, receptive or both) in the last six months. This is examined separately for respondents with regular and with casual partners (these groups overlap). Significant tests by χ^2 in cross-classifications, and by F test in analysis of variance. Probability levels less than .1 are shown.

Source: Connell et al. (1990).

low risk of HIV infection from casual partners. Very few men who described themselves as 'monogamous' engaged in dangerous anal practice with casual partners. But 'monogamy' was associated with a very high level of unprotected intercourse *within* the relationship. A finer breakdown by modality (not shown in Appendix 4A) reveals that a *majority* of 'monogamous' men engaged in receptive unprotected intercourse with their regular partners. It is clear that a substantial group in our sample act as though *being in a couple* removed the risk from sexual practice — or made them willing to run the risk (this is discussed in more detail in Chapter 11). This is an interesting and highly suggestive pattern. The findings for those with regular partners point to a restriction of sexual contacts among those who lead a riskier sex life within couples. This may be a deliberate strategy for many, to keep anal sex in their repertoire. For others, it may simply reflect that being in a regular relationship enables anal intercourse.

The second important pattern concerns gay community attachment measures. The measure of Sexual Engagement (SXE) showed opposite effects for the two measures of danger: sexual engagement in gay community was low for those who engaged in dangerous practice with regular partners, and high for those who engaged in dangerous practice with casual partners. Social Engagement was relatively low for those who engage in dangerous practice with either kind of partner — both findings were on the borderline of significance. Gay Community Involvement was low for those who engaged in dangerous practice with casual partners.

These findings point to the importance of distinguishing between different forms of involvement in gay community. Social and political involvement is likely to mean higher levels of support for a safe sex regime, while sexual engagement may not. We return to these issues in Chapter 9 where the findings are spelled out and their implications for HIV/AIDS prevention made clear.

To explore the settings of encounters where unsafe anal practice might be occurring, the 'danger' variable for casual partners was cross-classified with items about the use of particular venues. Five venues had been included in the inventory of sexual practices, and further questions were asked about (a) frequency of use and (b) level of enjoyment. In addition, in another part of the interview a set of questions was asked about (c) where a respondent sought sex partners. Results from the three groups of items were similar. Those for group (c) are shown in Table 6.3.

Men in the high danger group tended to make more use of certain sex-on-premises venues and enjoy them more. With saunas and beats

Table 6.3. Venues Where Sex Partners Are Sought* (n = 349)

	High danger (either or both modes)	Low danger (neither mode)	χ^2	df	p
	percentages				
Workplace	13.6	16.4	2.1	2	n.s.
Colleges	12.8	9.3	1.2	2	n.s.
Theatres	16.8	18.6	1.6	2	n.s.
Bars	73.6	72.5	1.3	2	n.s.
Saunas	56.8	42.8	7.0	2	.03
Discos	66.4	62.8	1.4	2	n.s.
Parties	72.8	74.3	1.9	2	n.s.
Beats	54.4	42.8	5.4	2	.07
Classified ads	18.4	13.8	2.8	2	n.s.
Bookshops	17.6	16.0	1.7	2	n.s.
Sex cinemas	8.0	3.7	3.9	2	n.s.
Prostitutes	5.6	4.5	1.8	2	n.s.
Gymnasia	10.4	19.0	6.1	2	.05
Pool, beaches	44.0	50.9	4.1	2	n.s.
Meetings	28.8	37.5	3.9	2	n.s.

Note: * Figures are percentages of persons who report using each venue, broken down by 'danger' in unprotected anal intercourse with casual partners (as defined in text).
Source: Connell *et al.* (1990).

in particular there was a difference between the high danger and the low danger group. It was in the settings where the making of casual sexual contacts was informally but definitely institutionalized that this difference showed through the three sets of items. No such differences between high danger and low danger groups appeared for less institutionalized settings, e.g., for the tendency to seek sex partners in workplaces, in bars, at parties. 'Finding partners' is not necessarily the same as having sex then and there.

To sum up the picture of dangerous practice that emerges from these data: unprotected anal intercourse was not a distinctive feature of a subgroup within this gay and bisexual population. It was, rather, a broadly distributed part of the repertoire. Our data point to two very different contexts where there was likely to be a higher than usual frequency of unprotected anal intercourse.

The first was indicated by the correlates of the Sexual Engagement scale and casual sex frequency, and by the data on venues. Read together, these point to a style of sexuality associated with multiple encounters in settings where casual sex is informally institutionalized. This is often spoken of as 'impersonal' sex, a misleading phrase. The more 'impersonal' contexts (prostitutes, parlours, classified advertisements) had low frequencies and did not show an association with the 'danger' variable. Indeed, we think of the style of sexuality in question as a form of community attachment, in the specific context of a *sexual community* (cf. D'Emilio, 1983) where anal intercourse has historically become a major focus of the social interchange. If this interpretation is broadly correct, the problem for prevention work is to find alternative forms of erotic attachment to gay social life.

The second key context of risky anal intercourse is within couple relationships. At the time of the survey nearly one-third of respondents were still engaging in unprotected intercourse with regular partners. More than half the men who described themselves as 'monogamous' did so. It is of course true that in an exclusive relationship between two people, both of whom are free of infection, no transmission of the virus can occur. But 'monogamous' does not always mean 'exclusive'. We have explored this issue in further life-history interviewing, and it appears that to some people 'monogamy' means a primary emotional commitment, not a completely exclusive sexual relationship. Even an exclusive relationship may not last. As we see in Chapter 11, there has been a considerable turnover in types of relationship over a five-year period. For instance, of those who describe themselves as having been 'monogamous' five years before, only 29 per cent describe themselves as 'monogamous' now, while 31 per cent of them have 'casual sex only' now. Practices of unsafe sex formed in a 'safe' relationship may be hard to change when the relationship is gone. On the other hand, it may also be possible that some men in HIV negative concordant regular relationships practise unprotected anal intercourse safely.

These connections between danger in practice and interpersonal and social milieu variables are noteworthy because they could well have been washed out by the powerful collective response to the HIV epidemic that has occurred. Sexual practice and sexual pleasure do not exactly coincide. It is at least conceivable that practice would have been homogenized by the impact of the epidemic. The findings here show that this had not happened at the date of the survey. Substantial differences in the organization of sexual practice remained and are connected with risk-taking.

There has been a move away from other unsafe practices, such as fisting the rectum; there has been an increased interest in oral-genital sex and sensuous touching and masturbation. Indeed, the latter practices, which are in the main safe, made up the bulk of our respondents' sexual activity. It was also these practices which men were more likely to engage in with their casual partners. Whether this was due to availability and accessibility, or to fear of HIV, it is impossible to tell from our data; possibly it was both.

Our specific findings on unsafe practices do *not* support a 'targeting' strategy where prevention/education work on unprotected anal intercourse would be directed to socially distinctive groups of men. For the bulk of the urban population it seems that broadly addressed programs are required. The content of broad-based programs needs to be focused on specific situations and judgments. The judgments about safety and risk reported in Table 6.1, for instance, are of concern. There is some risk for the insertive partner (see, for example, Kingsley *et al.*, 1987). Intercourse without ejaculation needs only a slight error of timing to turn into ejaculation inside — not an unusual occurrence, as Gold *et al.* (1989) have shown.

The fact that the main effects of the epidemic on sexuality appear to have been a slight contraction of the repertoire and a more limited choice of partners (Chapters 7 and 11), rather than a flowering of sexuality in new (safe) directions, points to the rather limited substitutability of practices. Yet our findings do suggest more constructive lines of development for preventive work. There are different sources of pleasure within sexuality. Preventive work might seek to build on the inherent gratifications of oral-genital sex (without ejaculation), a form of sex which is generally considered safe. The emotional satisfaction derived from communicative sex deserves attention. It is notable that sensuous touching, the practice that ranks highest for *emotionally satisfying*, is also the practice that gets near-universal endorsement as *very enjoyable*.

We are not suggesting that there is a separate group of communicative practices which can be substituted for others. Rather, we are suggesting that the communicative dimension inherent in *all* sexual practices be emphasized as a source of pleasure. Besides confirming current practice and eroticizing condoms, one might suggest that 'using condoms is your way of saying you care'. Such an approach would build on a notable feature of the HIV epidemic so far, the strength of gay men's collective response to it.

Some exceptions to the broad argument against 'targeted' programs should be noted. There are various indications of the need for a different kind of prevention work outside familiar gay communities. The newly sexual, of whatever age, also may need a distinctive approach. Older men will need support to sustain their change to safe practices. It is they who consistently nominate anal intercourse without condoms as the most satisfying sexual practice. These men, particularly those without a regular partner, are highly vulnerable. There is room for education about which partners gay men should use condoms with. Gay men may find it easier to sustain safe sex if they are given some autonomy with regard to condom use and thus can develop a sense of efficacy in the face of HIV. Men who are young and those who are marginalized in one way or another — lower income, few or no gay male friends, very little education — need special help. Although these men are more likely to have casual relationships only and are thus more likely to have less sex and/or to have oral-genital sex rather than anal sex, they are in need of more information about oral-genital sex. Many of these men have little if any sex because of their fear of HIV; such abstinence may be extremely difficult to sustain.

The argument made earlier in the chapter about the lack of long-term protection given by 'monogamy' seems to imply that prevention work should focus on the problems of relying on monogamy to prevent HIV transmission. Some medical researchers propose eliminating unprotected anal intercourse from all relationships: 'a prudent course would be to stop anal intercourse entirely' (Kingsley *et al.*, 1987: 348). Some men in the sample have moved very close to a 'total safe sex regime' in the sense of rigid obedience to all current safe sex rules. But not many have reached this state of grace; and the data suggest why.

The findings on enjoyment and satisfaction indicate that anal intercourse is one of the central practices in the gay/bisexual repertoire. It may even be argued — though this takes us beyond the current survey data — that for considerable numbers of men it has been experienced as a central part of being gay. So far as gay social life can be understood as a 'sexual community', this is a practice which has had a significant role in creating identities and social links. It is hardly surprising that statements of the personal importance of anal sex are consistently and strongly associated with frequency of practice. From this point of view, insisting on a total safe sex regime may be counter-productive. Over-rigid rules are impractical and invite blowouts: the net effect may be greater risk than a more moderate regime from the start.

Chapter 7

Changes in Response to HIV

From the moment AIDS was recognized as a sexually transmitted disease there were calls for changes in sexual behaviour directed especially at gay and bisexual men. Gay men were virtually identified with the disease in early media discussions and, in most of the Western capitalist countries (though not in the third world), were the group with the highest incidence of HIV infection. This remains the case in Australia.

What changes were taking place among Australian gay and bisexual men? Was the picture of men's sexuality in 1986/87, described in the previous chapter, very different from that in the years before the epidemic? Evidence referred to in Chapter 2 indicated that men were beginning to change their sexual practice prior to any awareness of the real threat of HIV in Australia. Had this change been augmented in response to HIV/AIDS? This was the central question addressed in the SAPA study. The other major question concerned the production of change. Had the educational initiatives of the gay communities and AIDS organizations influenced homosexually active men to change their sexual practice? Was the change a product of gay community educational efforts, or was it a function of contact with, and closeness to, the AIDS epidemic? What were the best predictors of change?

In the SAPA study we sought to know the following:

1   what kinds of practices were already changing, and what were not; this 'profile' of change would help gauge the success of prevention strategies so far and indicate where they might be focused next;

2   which social groups within the relevant population were changing relatively fast or relatively slowly and what group differences were there in the type of change that was prominent; if distinct

patterns were revealed, they would help focus prevention work more effectively; and

3   what indications could be gathered of the social and personal dynamics that produced the changes; this would help the design of effective educational material and programs, and, equally importantly, help avoid counter-productive moves.

The voices calling for change were diverse, and there was little consensus on the kind of change required: giving up homosexuality, giving up 'fast lane' lifestyles and anonymous sex, becoming monogamous, using condoms, or giving up anal sex. Despite the confusion, there are many indications that quite considerable changes in practice had occurred prior to our going into the field in 1986/87 and continued to occur long after. Researchers in the United States and Australia, for example, have reported similar pictures: declining average number of sexual partners (Feldman, 1985, in the United States) and sexual encounters (Frazer *et al.*, 1988, in Australia); high levels of change in sexual practices (Bennett and Petherbridge, 1986, in Australia); falling rates of HIV infection among samples of predominantly gay men (see Winkelstein *et al.*, 1987, for United States data, and Burcham *et al.*, 1989, for Australian data); and even a 'new sexual ethic' among gay men (William, 1984, in the United States).

More recently, studies indicate that men continue to make changes to their sexual behaviour in response to the threat of HIV: for example, in New York (Siegel *et al.*, 1988), in San Francisco (Ekstrand and Coates, 1990), in Chicago (Joseph *et al.*, 1990) and in England and Wales (Davies *et al.*, 1990; Hunt *et al.*, 1991). In the Western world there is mounting evidence indicating that many men who have sex with men have adopted safe sexual practices in response to the threat of AIDS.

The 'safe sex' campaigns for HIV/AIDS prevention can take some comfort from these findings, but how much? Hirsch and Enlow (1984) note several different patterns of personal response to the AIDS crisis in the United States: panicked rejection of sex (likely to reduce social support), denial of risk (possibly increasing exposure), and reduction of risky behaviour and support of community efforts against the disease. Kotarba and Lang (1986) also note contrasting responses by gay men to the epidemic. Bauman and Siegel (1987) document unrealistic optimism despite knowledge of safe sex rules and prevention tactics (such as washing) that are actually ineffective. Change, clearly, is not all of a piece and may not all be good. It is important to have a discriminating and detailed understanding of change in the face of the epidemic.

Patterns of change were explored in this study by means of two forced-choice inventories covering sexual practices, and a number of individual questions, both closed and open-ended. Research on changes in sexual behaviour, like some HIV/AIDS prevention publicity, often lumps change in personal relationships with change in sexual activities or techniques (e.g., the inventory of 'behavioural risk reduction' in Joseph *et al.*, 1987). We think it is crucial in HIV/AIDS education to make a clear distinction between (a) changes in the personal relationships that have a sexual aspect, that is, changes in the social 'framing' of emotional and sexual life such as the forming and the breaking of exclusive couples; and (b) changes in the way sexual pleasure is achieved, the sources and foci of sexual pleasure and the pattern of erotic interaction. Crudely stated, this is the distinction between whose bedroom you are in and what you do there. In designing the study we made a formal distinction between sexual relationships and sexual conduct or behaviour and developed a separate inventory for each. The eleven-item inventory on sexual relationships is shown in Table 7.2, and the fourteen-item inventory of sexual conduct is shown in Table 7.3.

We included in these inventories questions that reflected the then current practical concerns of AIDS prevention workers, debates about prevention in the media and technical literature, and what was known about change among gay and bisexual men in Australia. In addition to these inventories, we asked questions about changes in relationships, sexual conduct generally, condom use and like matters.

We stress again the importance of contextualizing sexual behaviour. As noted in Chapter 5, it is essential to place sexual behaviour in the context of the sexual relationship in which it takes place. When discussing changes in sexual practice, it is equally important to distinguish changes in sexual relationships from the changes that take place in sexual behaviours within those relationships. To change a particular practice requires a reshaping of the wider pattern of sexuality. This has not often been acknowledged or investigated in HIV/AIDS research.

Our respondents showed a strong awareness of change; a finding which parallels that of studies conducted in North America (e.g., Joseph *et al.*, 1987: 239). Asked, 'Do you think AIDS has changed your life?', only 11 per cent said 'no'. Invited to describe these changes, most painted a sombre picture of personal life and surrounding society: 'coming to terms with mortality; increase in stress in an already stressful environment; mood changes, depression, friends dying; and a loss of faith in society'; 'an element of fear in the gay community; negative public attitudes particularly from press and politicians — not all;

Table 7.1. Change in Relationship Status, for Respondents Aged 20 and Over (Figures within the table are frequencies.)

Now	Five years ago						
	None	Monogamous	Several	Relationship+ Casual*	Casual only	Total	Percentage
None	11	15	3	17	15	61	12
Monogamous	12	27	4	30	36	109	21
Several relationships	1	9	7	9	8	34	7
Relationship plus casual sex*	9	13	13	72	41	148	29
Casual sex only	10	29	6	38	72	155	30
Total	43	93	32	166	172	507	
Percentage	8	18	6	33	34		

Note: * This is a composite of three patterns: both partners in a relationship also having casual sex, or either having casual sex but not the other.
Source: Connell et al. (1989).

condoms.' Had this mood fuelled a revolution in sexual behaviour and relationships?

Changes in Sexual Relationships

We asked respondents to describe their sexual relationships at the time of the survey and about five years earlier, that is, before the AIDS crisis developed in Australia. Table 7.1 presents the cross-tabulation of these two questions for respondents aged 20 years and older (younger respondents being unlikely to have been in relationships five years before).

If one compares the totals, it is evident that there was a minor shift away from categories involving casual sex, but it was by no means as marked as the literature cited above would suggest. Overall responses from five years previously and the present were similar. It appears that the HIV epidemic had not resulted in a major shift in the overall framework of relationships. At the same time, as the interior of Table 7.1 shows, there was a great deal of individual movement between categories. A finer breakdown revealed that 112 of our over-20-year-old respondents had dropped casual sex over the last five years, but eighty-one had taken it up. These findings support Hirsch and Enlow's (1984) contention that the AIDS crisis results in diverse and even contradictory changes at the level of personal life.

We also asked the men in the survey whether they had made any

Table 7.2. Changes in Sexual Relationship Patterns in Response to Awareness of AIDS (overall percentages by item, n = 535)

		Yes	No	Never done	No response or don't know
1	Reducing the number of sexual partners	57	37	0	6
2	Avoiding sex with certain individuals	56	37	1	6
3	Cutting down on sex generally	47	48	0	5
4	Changing the sort of men I pick up	36	54	2	8
5	Avoiding sex with people who are AB+*	33	47	8	12
6	Changing the places I pick men up	31	58	2	8
7	Avoiding sex with prostitutes	20	10	63	7
8	Becoming monogamous	19	72	3	6
9	Asking my partner to become monogamous	18	64	5	14
10	Avoiding sex with people whose AB* status I don't know	16	70	5	9
11	Avoiding sex with people who are AB-*	7	72	6	15

Note: * Refer to HIV antibody (blood) test results.
Source: Connell *et al.* (1989).

changes *in response* to HIV and AIDS. The data derived from two questions — the first, 'For you, has awareness of AIDS led you to make any changes to your sexual relations?', also indicated that men had changed their sexual practice. These data are retrospective reports on change. We did, however, reinterview some of the men in 1991; the reported changes were echoed in the changes made between 1986/87 and 1991 (Kippax *et al.*, 1993). We will return to this follow-up study later in this chapter and in Chapter 11.

As shown in Table 7.2, the men, when surveyed in 1986/87, reported that they had made changes to their sexual relationships. The eleven items are listed in order of the level of reported change. The most common responses were those of reduced overall sexual contact (items 1 and 3) and being more particular about the choice of partner (items 2, 4 and 5). Change in the structure of relationships was much less pronounced; these answers reinforced the message of Table 7.1. There was no stampede into monogamy, though a significant minority moved down this path.

Changes in Sexual Behaviour

The men in our study also reported that they had made changes to their sexual behaviours within their relationships. In response to the

Table 7.3. Changes in Specific Sexual Practices (overall percentages by item).

	Never done	Stopped	Do it less	About same	Do it more	Started	No response
				(percentages)			
Using condoms	11	1	0.2	4	29	42	14
'Safe sex' with casual partners	3	2	3	8	40	28	14
'Safe sex' with regular partners	7	2	1	20	29	19	22
Sensuous touching, massage	1	0.2	1	42	43	0.4	13
Mutual masturbation	2	1	1	43	39	1	13
Masturbating alone	0.4	0.4	3	64	19	0	13
Reading/watching porn	5	1	4	64	12	1	13
SM — without drawing blood	80	5	1	1	0	0.2	13
Fisting	56	16	8	6	1	1	14
'Unsafe sex' with regular partners	7	34	19	16	1	0	22
Watersports	66	10	6	4	0	1	13
'Unsafe sex' with casual partners	8	52	24	2	0	0.4	14
SM — which draws blood	80	5	1	1	0	0.2	13
Scat	84	2	1	0	0	0.2	13

Note: No responses are mainly respondents who replied, 'No changes at all' to a filter question, 'Has your awareness of AIDS led you to make any changes in your sexual activities?'
Source: Connell *et al.* (1989).

question, 'For you, has awareness of AIDS led you to make any changes in your sexual activities?', 87 per cent of the men reported that they had made some changes. Table 7.3 shows responses to the inventory of specific practices, again listing the items in order of popularity.

While change in sexual behaviour was widespread, it was highly discriminating. The practices that had increased were essentially those described as 'safe sex'. The nuances are also noteworthy. For instance, there was a higher rate of adopting safe sex practices with casual rather than regular partners and a higher rate of stopping unsafe sex with casual partners. But a significant number of men had not moved towards safer sexual contact within a regular relationship.

The lower half of Table 7.3 shows forms of sexual conduct that had been reduced and in some cases almost entirely dropped. There seem to be two different patterns here. The first is the safe sex message again, but inverted. It is notable that fisting was being given up; a majority of those who had ever engaged in fisting reported that they had stopped. The second pattern emerged with practices that were in decline despite the fact that they were not (or not necessarily) unsafe with regard to HIV transmission. These items include sado-masochistic practices ('SM'), urolagnia ('water-sports'), and sex with faeces ('scat'). In all cases the participation rate was low to start with (see the 'never done' column) and had become lower. There seems to be an interplay here between rational fear of HIV and stigmatization of esoteric or more adventurous sexual practices.

The overall picture shows a contracting sexual repertoire. There is no doubt that men perceived that they had changed their sexual behaviour in response to the threat of HIV. There was less sex, less esoteric sex, and there were fewer partners. If there is a 'new sexual ethic', as William (1984) suggested, there is also a newly scaled-down sex life. Only 24 per cent of our sample described themselves as 'very happy' with the changes in their sex life; an equal number were at best 'ambivalent'. Responses were on the whole sombre.

An Analysis of Change

In line with the above descriptive analysis, and as summarized in Chapter 4, the items that measured responses to change in sexual practice formed two scales. The first measured relationship change (RC). Changing one's pattern of relationships is advocated by certain HIV prevention strategists, those who emphasize monogamy, and by the conservative political and religious commentators who urge gay men to celibacy. The construction of the Relationship Change (RC) scale shows that there was an identifiable response of this kind among our respondents.

The second measured changes to sexual practice. These items were combined in such a way as to provide a measure of the degree to which the men had adopted safe sexual behaviours (AS). The safe sex strategy has been advocated in prevention campaigns that consider it important to be pro-sex and positive about being gay. The construction of the Adopting Safe Sex (AS) scale shows that this, too, was an identifiable response among our respondents.

Our measures, therefore, distinguish these two types of change: the first scale, RC, measures changes in the nature of the relationships such as a move into monogamy or the reduction of the number of casual sexual partners; the second scale, AS, measures actual changes in sexual activities such as the use of condoms and the foregoing of fisting.

Having demonstrated that there was change, our interest shifted to identifying what enabled and produced the changes described. We shall describe the outcome of our analysis here and in the remainder of the book concentrate on the best predictors of the changes we documented — attachment to gay community and informed social support.

In our analysis of change, these two scales, AS and RC, became our dependent measures. The independent measures we included in the analysis were those which we thought might give us some insight into the production of the change in sexual practice. As discussed in Chapters 1 and 3, as well as including variables which are typical of many explanatory models, such as knowledge of and attitudes towards the behaviours in question, we also included milieu variables which capture the social and cultural context of the behaviours, and others which capture the interpersonal context. The independent measures included in our explanatory model were:

a number of social descriptors — age, religion, country of origin, income, labour force status, occupation and educational level achieved;

a number of milieu variables — three scales of gay community attachment and engagement which measured degree of Sexual Engagement (SXE) in gay community, Social Engagement (SCE) and cultural and political Gay Community Involvement (GCI); one scale of degree of Contact with the Epidemic (CE); a single item based on place of residence which we called Locale, and a single item of HIV serostatus, Test Status;

measures of accuracy of information and beliefs about HIV and AIDS — two scales measuring accuracy of Knowledge of Safe Sex (KSS) and Knowledge of Unsafe Sex (KUS); one scale measuring General Issues (GI) concerning AIDS; and another measuring Awareness of AIDS Pamphlets (PA); and

measures of current sexual practice and relationship status — three scales measuring the variety of current sexual practice, the Oral/Tactile Practice (OTP), Essentially Anal Practice (EAP) and the Infrequent Esoteric Practice (IEP) scales, and a single item which measured Relationship Status.

A multiple regression analysis was used to examine the relationship between the dependent and independent variables and to uncover the best predictors of the adoption of safe sexual practice (AS) and relationship change (RC). The variables included in the multiple regression were those which were significant in univariate analyses. These were the social descriptor variables, age and education; the milieu measures, the Locale and Test Status items, the Contact with the Epidemic scale and the three gay community attachment scales, GCI, SCE, SXE; and the knowledge scales, KSS, KUS, GI and PA. The sexual practice scales, OTP, EAP and IEP, as well as relationship status were also included. A full account of the analysis is given in Connell *et al.* (1989) and in Kippax *et al.* (1992), and a detailed analysis of the statistical relationship between contact with the epidemic, place of residence and the three measures of attachment to gay community in relation to changes in sexual practice is found in Crawford, Kippax and Dowsett (1990).

Adoption of Safe Sex

The variables which contributed most to sexual behaviour change (AS) were two of the gay community attachment scales, Sexual Engagement (SXE) and Social Engagement (SCE), and Locale. Another variable of some importance was knowledge of 'unsafe' sex, KUS. The nature of sexual relationship and sexual practice were also implicated, but these may be simply functions of change as well as predictors of it (see Table 7.4).

In the full model, the variables accounted for 23.2 per cent of the variance in the adoption of safe sex. The social descriptor variables when fitted alone accounted for 1.5 per cent, the milieu variables for 15.2 per cent and the knowledge variables for 5.8 per cent. Clearly, the milieu variables, especially the gay community attachment measures, were the most important set. What the analysis showed was that place of residence and attachment to gay community, particularly Sexual Engagement and, to a lesser extent, Social Engagement, were most important for change in sexual behaviour. The greater the engagement, the greater the change.

An accurate knowledge of 'unsafe' sexual practice contributed to change to 'safe' sexual behaviour. Education contributed a small amount to change; men with more years of education were more likely to have changed their practice in the direction of 'safe' sex than men with fewer years of education. Those in monogamous relationships had changed least, while those in several relationships had changed most. Also, men who engaged in a wide variety of oral and tactile sexual practices had changed most. It is likely that the significant relationships between sexual relationship status and sexual practice, on the one hand, and change in sexual practice, on the other, were a result of a move to these 'safe' sexual practices by the men surveyed rather than predictors of that change.

Table 7.4. Regression Model: Adoption of Safe Sex

Variable	Full model			Reduced model			
	r	R^2 (%)	% var fitted last	Regression coefficients raw	standard	t	p	% var fitted last
Age	−.033	0.1	0.3					
Education	.111	1.2	0.9	.193	.113	2.79	.005	1.2
None				.460	.224	1.56	.119	
Monogamous				−.650	−.315	−2.50	.013	
Several		7.8	2.6	.715	.348	2.07	.039	2.8
Regular plus (compared with casual only)				.064	.031	0.27	.784	
SXE	.337	11.3	2.7	.098	.215	4.35	.000	2.9
SCE	.196	3.8	0.4	.081	.097	2.25	.025	1.0
GCI	.185	3.4	0.1					
Northern suburbs				.310	.151	0.99	.323	
Outer Sydney				−.183	−.089	−0.69	.493	
Extra-metropolitan		3.4	0.7	−.480	−.234	−1.96	.050	0.9
Canberra (compared with Inner Sydney)				−.076	−.037	−0.24	.811	
CE	.162	2.6	0.5	.121	.063	1.44	.150	0.1
KSS	.016	0.0	0.0					
KUS	.119	1.4	1.4	.113	.123	3.09	.002	1.4
KSP	.028	0.1	0.1					
GI	.136	1.8	0.5					
PA	.115	1.3	0.2					
Positive				.518	.253	1.91	.057	
Negative (compared with untested)		1.7	0.5	.164	.080	0.84	.402	0.6
IEP	.036	0.1	0.6	−.133	−.096	−2.25	.025	0.6
EAP	.092	0.8	0.0					
OTP	.161	2.6	0.7	.194	.134	2.89	.004	1.0
	R^2 = 23.05%				R^2 = 21.8%			

Source: Kippax *et al.* (1992).

The importance of gay community attachment and place of residence was indicated by the following: that those who live in Extra-metropolitan NSW had changed least when compared with men who live in Inner Sydney. This relationship holds over and above gay community attachment. On the other hand, Contact with the Epidemic was not important once the gay community attachment and Locale variables were taken into account. Gay community attachment and place of residence were important explanatory concepts over and above their relationship with Contact with the Epidemic.

Relationship Change

A similar regression was carried out with relationship change as the dependent variable. The reduced model showed that knowledge of 'safe' sex (KSS) and place of residence as measured by Locale were important variables with regard to relationship change, as was education level. Measures of attachment to gay community were not strongly related to relationship change; Sexual Engagement in gay community (SXE) was marginally significant (see Table 7.5).

The full model accounted for 14.2 per cent of the variance and the reduced model for 10.4 per cent (12.1 per cent if sexual relationship status is included). The analysis indicated that men with little accurate knowledge of 'safe' sex and with little education were more likely to change their relationship status than others. It is almost as though they had changed their relationship status because they were not sure which sexual practices were 'safe'. Gay community attachment was of little importance, while place of residence had some impact on relationship change. Men in Extra-metropolitan NSW and men in the Northern suburbs of Sydney, when compared with men in Inner Sydney, were most likely to have changed their sexual relationships towards monogamy and celibacy.

Conclusions

The men surveyed in the SAPA study in 1986/87 reported that since the advent of AIDS, they had adopted a wide range of strategies that they believed enabled them to avoid transmitting HIV and avoid HIV infection. Such strategies included the use of condoms for anal intercourse, the exclusion of anal intercourse from men's sexual repertoires, the foregoing of anal intercourse with casual partners, care in selection of partners, and moves to monogamy and even celibacy.

In general, gay community attachment and place of residence were the most important predictors of change. These data indicate the importance of informed social support. Gay community and place of residence are implicated in the relationship between knowledge and change. Knowledge of 'safe' sex, something that to some extent only the gay communities dealt with in their media and educational

Table 7.5. *Regression Model: Relationship Change*

Variable	r	R^2 (%)	% var fitted last	Reduced model		t	p	% var fitted last
				Regression coefficients				
				raw	standard			
Age	.011	0.0	0.0					
Education	−.132	1.7	0.9	−.257	−.115	−2.73	.007	1.3
None								
Monogamous								
Several		2.5	0.9					
Regular plus (compared with casual only)								
SXE	−.070	0.5	0.8	−.048	−.080	−1.92	.055	0.6
SCE	−.043	0.2	0.0					
GCI	−.059	0.3	0.0					
Northern suburbs				.906	.336	2.15	.032	
Outer Sydney				.065	.024	0.18	.865	
Extra-metropolitan			2.2	.967	.358	2.95	.003	2.8
Canberra (compared with Inner Sydney)				−.404	−.150	−0.94	.346	
CE	.023	0.1	0.2					
KSS	−.244	6.0	1.5	−.170	−.207	−4.89	.000	4.1
KUS	.155	2.4	0.1					
KSP	−.133	1.8	0.2					
GI	.106	1.1	0.0					
PA	−.083	0.7	0.1					
Positive								
Negative (compared with untested)		0.7	0.9					
IEP	.027	0.1	0.1					
EAP	.043	0.2	0.3					
OTP	−.067	0.4	0.4					
			$R^2 = 14.2\%$				$R^2 = 10.4\%$	

Note: If sexual relationships are included, SXE is not significant, and reduced model $R^2 = 12.1\%$.
Source: Kippax *et al.* (1992).

campaigns, is related to change. Men who did not know what constitutes 'safe' sex were the ones most likely to change their relationship status, while men who had the more accurate information about what is 'unsafe' were most likely to change their sexual practice. In order to move to 'safe' sexual practice, knowledge of what is 'safe' is also needed.

Contact with the epidemic is important, but its impact on change is mediated by gay community attachment. If there is no gay community attachment, then contact with the epidemic works towards sexual behaviour change. Where attachment to gay community is reasonably strong, however, contact with the epidemic adds little by way of a contribution to change. Test result is, in general, unimportant.

Educators who stress the need to address communities from the point of view of the communities themselves are correct. The sexually confident, well educated gay men, who live in Sydney or Canberra, who are sexually and socially engaged with gay community, and who are well informed about 'safe' and 'unsafe' sex, are more likely to have changed their sexual behaviour than homosexually active men who are not attached to gay community, who live in extra-metropolitan NSW, who have had little contact with the epidemic and are unsure of what is 'safe'. These men are to some degree more likely than the former to change the nature of their sexual relationships in order to protect themselves from HIV infection. It is important to note, however, that there are not two separate identifiable groups of men — one group who change their sexual behaviour, the other who change the nature of their relationships. Some men have changed both their sexual practice and the nature of their relationships; others have changed little with regard to either; and other men have modified aspects of both their sexual behaviour and their relationships (Connell *et al.*, 1989). Both strategies involve risk; 'safe' sex may be difficult to sustain over a period of time and relationship changes do not necessarily protect one from infection. With regard to the latter point, figures suggest that, at the time of the survey, there was an increase in the number of men in regular relationships who are becoming infected (Tindall *et al.*, 1989).

It is evident that education campaigns should continue to be informed by gay communities and that the men who perhaps are most at risk are those who are not reached by gay community campaigns. Men who for whatever reason are separate from any form of attachment to gay community need special attention; many of these men appear not to be sure about the sexual practices in which they can safely engage with virtually no risk of HIV infection.

Knowledge of safe and unsafe sexual practices, attachment to gay community and place of residence are the most important predictors of changes in sexual practice. Details of the ways in which HIV-related information is accessed and the role of gay community attachment in the adoption of safe sexual practice are given in Chapters 8 and 9.

Chapter 8

HIV-related Information

Much has been said of the relationship between the information and knowledge that people possess about the transmission of HIV and subsequent changes in their behaviour. The Health Belief Model (Becker, 1974; Becker and Joseph, 1988) and the Theory of Reasoned Action (Fishbein and Ajzen, 1975; Fishbein and Middlestadt, 1989) have been applied to the problem of the primary prevention of AIDS. Both models are, on the whole, somewhat simplistic. Although they have been extended and elaborated, the latter in the direction of incorporating normative beliefs, they both focus on the individual as the seat of change and both assume a linear movement — from knowledge, to attitude, to intention, to behaviour change. Fishbein and Middlestadt conclude that

> . . . in order to change or reinforce a given behaviour in a given population effectively, we must first determine whether the behavior is under attitudinal or normative control *in that population*, and we must identify the salient beliefs underlying the attitude or subjective norm. That is, we should be aware of what the members of that population already know about performing the behavior. . . . (1989: 109; their emphasis)

Both models have been criticized for their failure to account for sexual behaviour change, or lack of it, in the context of HIV/AIDS (see Kippax and Crawford, in press). Kirscht and Joseph (1989), for example, point to the importance of the interpretation that individuals make of their own behaviour. But more than this is needed to give an adequate account of how HIV-related information is appropriated. The meanings in terms of which individuals interpret their own and others' behaviour and the normative beliefs of particular populations, cultural and subcultural norms, are produced *collectively* in efforts to make sense of the AIDS epidemic. Understandings are reached via media representations of HIV/AIDS, medical findings and pronouncements, legal, church and other institutional responses to the issues surrounding HIV and AIDS, government-sponsored educational messages and campaigns, community responses and interpersonal interactions. Meanings are also reached within the prevailing normative structures and discourses which produce and govern sexual practice and sexuality: discourses which underpin beliefs about men's and women's biological make-up, gender differences, love and commitment.

The first reports about AIDS appeared in Australia in 1981 and 1982; these reports focused on the puzzling illness that was affecting gay men in the United States. The early medical reports focused on multiple partners, anal sex and the use of drugs in sex as possible causes of the disease — an implicit connection between disease and deviance (see Shilts, 1988). A moralism was evident in many of the early epidemiological reports (e.g., Goedert, 1987). The notion of 'risk group' was built into the ways in which epidemiological data were categorized and reported (see Chapter 2).

The media, like the general public, turned to the medical profession for information about AIDS and the ways in which HIV is transmitted and can be avoided. With some exceptions the mainstream media adopted a moralistic attitude and, with the exception of 'innocent victims' who had been infected via the blood supply, scapegoated those who were unfortunate enough to be among those infected early. The mainstream media provided a supply of ready-made opinions which passed as knowledge: 'Modern mass communications, moulded after industrial production, spread a whole system of stereotypes which, while still being fundamentally "ununderstandable" to the individual, allow him at any moment to appear as being up to date and "knowing all about it" ' (Adorno *et al.*, 1950: 665).

In Australia the media in the early years represented AIDS as a plague in which heterosexuals are threatened by deviant others (Lupton, 1991a, 1991b; Tulloch, 1989). Here, in the United States and Great Britain, AIDS was associated with two highly stigmatized groups — homosexuals and intravenous drug users. More generally, promiscuity was and continues to be targeted as a risky practice (Brandt, 1988; Hart, 1985; Horton and Aggleton, 1989; Markova and Wilkie, 1987; Sontag, 1988; Watney, 1987).

Since then the mainstream and gay press, in somewhat different ways, have informed the public about AIDS, HIV and safe sex. The former has focused on the dangers associated with various practices, while the latter also noted ways in which sex could be made safe. In Chapter 2 we described the ways in which the gay community educated its constituency with regard to HIV transmission. We also described the ways in which the Commonwealth and state governments funded gay community and other non-government AIDS organizations to enable them to continue and extend the preventive campaigns they had already begun.

In 1987 the Commonwealth government also launched its first national campaign. The campaign, although criticized by many, did not focus on risk groups but rather targeted practices which placed one at risk of HIV. From about 1987 onwards education campaigns, both within and outside the gay community, informed people of the issues surrounding the transmission of HIV and ways of dealing with and preventing the spread of the virus. These gay community and government-sponsored education campaigns were in the main at odds with the early media reporting. Their focus was practice, both sexual and drug use, and ways in which HIV transmission could be avoided. Condoms, other forms of safe sex practice, and non-sharing of needles and syringes were central to the educational message.

Evidence, both in Australia (Anns, 1987; McCamish, 1987; Millan and Ross, 1987; Sinnott and Todd, 1987; Carr, 1988) and in the United States of America (Coates, Temoshok and Mandel, 1984; McCusick, Horstman and Coates, 1985; Emmons *et al.*, 1986; Joseph *et al.*, 1987a, 1987b; Strunin and Hingson, 1987; and Carr's report on the Third International AIDS conference, Carr, 1987) indicates that the type and accuracy of knowledge about HIV/AIDS is a function of a number of the factors outlined above. These studies show that some people are well informed, while others are not; and the relationship between knowledge and behaviour change is a complex one. DiClemente, Zorn and Temoshok (1987) found marked variability in knowledge across informational items, and their data indicated that proximity to an AIDS epicentre is of great importance to accuracy of knowledge of HIV. Sherr (1987), evaluating the impact of a British government health education campaign, found that those from 'higher-risk' groups were more likely to notice and read the campaign material then those from 'lower-risk' groups. The campaign, however, had no effect on correcting misconceptions, and attitudes and behaviour were unaltered.

The SAPA study, too, investigated the amount and type of information possessed by gay and bisexual men about HIV/AIDS issues, and the major sources of that information. There were two major foci:

the first was to explore the manner in which men came to understand issues of HIV transmission and AIDS and to examine the factors implicated in the formation of the men's beliefs and knowledge; the second was to investigate the relationship between such knowledge and changes in sexual practice.

Profile of Knowledge and Doubt

The questionnaire included groups of items concerned with knowledge and opinion. Two of these dealt with knowledge about the safety or riskiness of a variety of social and sexual practices, while the third focused on general issues related to HIV and AIDS. The first group listed twelve items of social behaviours (such as sharing a bath, sharing a razor) which respondents were asked to rate for safety. The second group listed seventeen items of general information, such as 'Someone could pass on AIDS while appearing very healthy.' The largest group of items was an inventory of thirty-one sexual practices which respondents were asked to rate for safety or risk 'with respect to passing on the AIDS virus'. As only the last group of items, those dealing with the safety or otherwise of a number of sexual practices, was significantly related to change, only these items will be discussed in detail.

With regard to the social practices, most of the men correctly judged the safety of these practices. There were high levels of confidence about most of these; the majority of respondents perceived these practices as 'very safe', although, again, small minorities were extremely cautious. Two items were rated differently from the others; 'sharing a razor' and 'sharing a toothbrush', the ones most likely to involve exchange of body fluids. In both cases 43 per cent of respondents estimated that these behaviours constituted a 'small risk'.

As for the general information items, the men were well acquainted with the broader issues surrounding the transmission of HIV, but less sure of immunological matters, for example, whether there would soon be a vaccine, or whether repeated occurrences of sexually transmitted diseases made one more vulnerable to HIV.

Table 8.1 presents the judged safety of a selection of the sexual practice items. There are many points of interest in this table. Practices widely considered to be 'very safe' by the men in the sample included dry kissing, mutual masturbation, and sensuous touching (also variants of this omitted from Table 8.1 to save space). Nevertheless, a small minority perceived risk even in these practices. A majority also perceived

Table 8.1. Judgments of Safety/Risk of Sexual Practices[a] (n = 535)

Sexual practice	Judgments (percentage of respondents)			
	'Very safe'	'Small risk'	'Not at all safe'	'Don't know'/'unsure'
1 Sensuous touching	95	5	0	0
2 Dry kissing	83	12	1	1
3 Wet/deep kissing	39	54	4	3
4 Mutual masturbation	93	6	1	0
5 Cock rings[b]	82	10	4	3
6 S/M dom/bond no blood	70	20	5	5
7 Anal intercourse with condom (insertive)	48	50	1	1
8 (receptive)	40	57	3	0
9 Watersports (giving)	45	25	21	9
10 (receptive)	31	33	25	10
11 Watersports in the mouth (giving)	28	21	41	10
12 (receptive)	8	26	55	11
13 Scat[b]	5	17	63	14
14 Fingerfucking (insertive)	37	43	16	4
15 (receptive)	35	44	18	4
16 Oral-genital no semen (insertive)	34	56	9	2
17 (receptive)	23	64	12	1
18 Fisting (insertive)	22	35	37	6
19 (receptive)	18	31	45	6
20 Oral-anal contact (insertive)	7	30	60	4
21 (receptive)	16	37	42	5
22 Dildo/toy (insertive[b])	55	30	12	2
23 (receptive[b])	43	37	17	2
24 Oral-genital with semen (insertive)	19	36	44	2
25 (receptive)	4	30	65	1
26 Anal intercourse no ejaculation (insertive)	11	55	33	1
27 (receptive)	9	49	42	1
28 Anal intercourse no condom (insertive)	2	24	74	1
29 (receptive)	1	5	94	0
30 S/M dom/bond with blood (giving[b])	19	21	55	5
31 (receptive[b])	10	22	64	4

Notes: a Responses coded as correct were:
    'Very safe' — items 1–17 inclusive
    'Small risk' or 'not at all safe' — items 18–23 inclusive
    'Not at all safe' — items 24–31 inclusive.
    All other responses were coded as incorrect.
  b Items 5, 13, 22, 23, 30 and 31 do not scale.
    Items 1, 2, 3, 4, 6, 7, 8, 9, 10, 11, 12, 14, 15, 16 and 17 form KSS scale.
    Items 18, 19, 20, 21, 24, 25, 26, 27, 28 and 29 form KUS scale.
Source: Kippax *et al.* (1990).

sado-masochistic practices (without blood) and the use of cock rings as 'very safe', but a sizeable minority believed there was a 'small risk' associated with these practices. Conversely, practices considered 'not at all safe' by the men surveyed included anal intercourse without condoms, oral-anal contact (particularly insertive), receiving urine in the mouth 'water sports', sexual play with faeces 'scat', oral-genital contact involving semen exchange (particularly receptive), and sado-masochistic practices which draw blood.

A considerable number of sexual practices did not fall into either of these two categories. With regard to these practices, which included wet kissing, oral-genital contact without semen exchange, watersports other than those involving urine in the mouth, fist 'fisting' and finger 'fingerfucking' in the rectum, and the use of dildos, either a majority of the respondents perceived these sexual practices as 'small risk' practices or the sample was divided over the perception of risk. As well, respondents were relatively unsure of the safety of certain practices: those involving oral-anal contact and sado-masochism with blood, and watersports, fisting and scat received a large number of 'don't know' responses. As might be expected, there is an overlap between these practices and those, described above, about which there was a spread of opinion among the respondents.

Several conclusions may be drawn from these three sets of items which tap information about the safety of a variety of sexual and social practices. First, a broad distinction was made by the men between activities (both sexual and social) that involve blood, semen or saliva and activities in which there is little likelihood of the exchange of body fluids. The items on which there was most agreement are those where there is an unequivocal presence or absence of blood, semen or saliva. There was less certainty and far greater variance with respect to practices where blood, semen or saliva *may* be present — even social practices like sharing a toothbrush or razor were regarded by many as risky. The sample as a whole seemed reasonably well informed about the principal message of AIDS education, the avoidance of body fluids exchange.

Second, there were significant areas of doubt, as evidenced by the number of 'don't know' responses, and/or disagreement among the respondents. For example, the sample was unsure about the safety of the frequently practised forms of oral-genital contact. As well, the sample was uncertain of the safety of some practices which are not objectively risky in terms of HIV transmission (on medical knowledge now and at the time) but which are distinctly minority practices, such as some forms of water sports and scat.

The Question of Accuracy

At the time the responses to the questionnaire were coded, in mid-1987, medical opinion was divided with respect to some of the practices. When we coded the responses for accuracy, we turned to the AIDS Council of New South Wales, and they advised us of their assessment of the safety or risk of HIV transmission of the various practices — sexual and social. The coding for accuracy, as shown in Table 8.1, was based on this advice, and that is what the term 'accuracy' means in this book.

If the items are scored for accuracy, then the data indicate that AIDS education efforts have had considerable success in disseminating information about some aspects of the epidemic. In the sample of men surveyed there was very widespread understanding that anal intercourse without condoms is dangerous; that some other sexual practices like sensuous touching are quite safe; and that most ordinary social contacts are safe. It is equally true, however, that there were some areas of concern. For example, with regard to oral-genital sex, an almost universal practice among the men (see Chapter 5), there was a great deal of disagreement and doubt.

One Meaning or More?

We had hypothesized that there would be one factor — a factor which measured accuracy — and that the men in the sample could be given a score assessing their knowledge of the safety of practices with regard to HIV transmission. The items did not scale or form a homogeneous group; there was not a single measure of knowledge. The items contain different meanings for the respondents.

Certain sets of items did scale, however. The items tapping information about the safety of sexual practice fell into two main clusters: one included practices currently held by the medical profession to be safe, and the other included practices currently thought to be risky (see Table 8.2). These two scales, which we called Knowledge of Safe Sex (KSS) and Knowledge of Unsafe Sex (KUS), form reliable scales with good face validity.

KSS is a fifteen-item scale which measures the accuracy of knowledge of 'safe' (deemed so by medical opinion at the time of the survey) sexual practices. It should be noted that the scale does not include 'scat', or the use of cock rings and dildos, as these items did not scale. The higher the scale score, the more accurate was the respondent's

Table 8.2. Two Information Scales, KSS, KUS, and their Scale Characteristics

| KSS | | KUS | |
Item	Item-total correlation	Item	Item-total correlation
1	0.17	18	0.39
2	0.33	19	0.37
3	0.31	20	0.31
4	0.23	21	0.37
6	0.35	24	0.41
7	0.42	25	0.34
8	0.33	26	0.45
9	0.56	27	0.36
10	0.50	28	0.38
11	0.45	29	0.21
12	0.31		
14	0.57		alpha = 0.70
15	0.54		
16	0.50		
17	0.43		
	alpha = 0.80		

Source: Kippax et al. (1990).

knowledge of safe sex practices. Individual scores ranged from 0 to 15. The mean KSS score of 7.10 and standard deviation of 3.29 indicated, in general, that knowledge of safe sex practice was moderate (see Tables 8.1 and 8.2). The reliability of this scale was 0.80 as measured by Cronbach's alpha.

KUS is a ten-item scale which measures the accuracy of knowledge of unsafe practices (see Tables 8.1 and 8.2). It should be noted that the KUS scale does not include sado-masochistic practices which draw blood as these items did not scale. As with the above scales, the higher the scale score, the more accurate was the respondent's knowledge of risky sex practices. The range of KUS was from 0 to 10, the mean scale score was 6.68, and there was a standard deviation of 2.25, indicating a moderate knowledge of unsafe practices. The reliability of this scale (Cronbach's alpha) was 0.70.

Meanings of 'Safe' and 'Risky'

These two scales were related to each other in a somewhat surprising way: KSS and KUS were strongly and *negatively* related, r = −0.51: accuracy of information about safe sex was negatively related to accuracy of information about risky sex.

Table 8.3, which shows the relationship between individual scores on KSS and KUS, provided some insight into this unusual relationship

Table 8.3.   Relationship between Respondents' Scores on KSS and KUS

		KUS score	Percentage of respondents	
		Low (0–5)	High (6–10)	Total
KSS score				
	Low (0–7)	6.8	50.0	56.8
	High (8–15)	21.4	21.8	43.2
	Total	28.2	71.8	100.0

Source: Kippax *et al.* (1990).

between the accuracy of knowledge about 'safe' and 'unsafe' sexual practices. Although there was only a small proportion of men who had inaccurate knowledge of both 'safe' and 'unsafe' practices (7 per cent), and a larger proportion who had a moderately accurate knowledge of both 'safe' and 'unsafe' practices (22 per cent), there were relatively large proportions of men who, at one and the same time, were both reasonably well informed about 'unsafe' practices and not very well informed about 'safe' practices (50 per cent) and vice versa (21 per cent). As the mean scores on the KSS and KUS indicate, men were likely to be marginally better informed about 'unsafe' sex than 'safe' sex.

These data indicated that most gay and bisexual men possessed a moderate, but somewhat uneven, knowledge of the safety of sexual practices. There are a number of possible interpretations of this unevenness in knowledge. As noted above, mainstream media until 1987 had concentrated on AIDS which they linked to unsafe practices such as anal intercourse. The gay press, on the other hand, as well as informing its readers about unsafe practices also directed its audience (men in the gay communities) to practices that were considered safe. The wider distribution of the mainstream media may explain the finding that a large number of the men (50 per cent) had a 'high' score with regard to 'unsafe' sexual practices and a 'low' score with regard to practices which we classified as 'safe'.

As noted above, the men in the sample were less sure of sexual activities where the exchange of body fluids is equivocal or uncertain. Practices which involved oral-genital and anal-oral contact have received little attention and as a result many respondents were confused as to their safety or otherwise. Some men distinguished between oral-genital sex which involves ejaculation and that which does not, while others rated all forms of oral-genital sex as risky or all forms of oral-genital sex as safe. This tendency on the part of some men either to overestimate or to underestimate the risk of sexual practices was a general one; it was apparent in men's judgments of almost all practices but particularly those of uncertain risk status. In general, however, erring on the side of caution was more common than errors in the other direction; this accounts for the finding that men knew more about 'unsafe' practice than they knew about 'safe'.

Contexts of the Formation of Judgments

We now turn to an examination of the factors which influence the knowledge possessed by the men in the study. The literature reviewed above indicates that social factors such as place of residence, attachment to the gay community, identification with at-risk populations, mediate the ways in which information is received.

Both univariate and multivariate analyses were carried out to assess the impact of a number of social descriptors on the accuracy of information possessed by the men in the sample. Generally, the results indicated that the accuracy of judgments of 'safe' sexual practices, as measured by KSS, was unrelated to social descriptors. The exception was education; there was a slight trend for the more highly educated to have more accurate information about 'safe' sexual practices. Accuracy with regard to 'safe' sexual practices was unrelated to age, national origin, income, occupation, labour force status and religion. There was no relationship between any of these social descriptors and the accuracy of judgments of 'unsafe' sexual practices as measured by the KUS scale. Knowledge about safe and unsafe practices was widespread and uniform, at least with respect to these social descriptors.

Factors which may give some indication of the impact of social context on the ways in which information is taken up were also investigated. Those selected for discussion here are:

place of residence or locale: the sample was divided between those who lived in the Inner Sydney suburbs (most closely associated with gay community), Northern Sydney suburbs, Outer Sydney suburbs, Extra-metropolitan towns and centres in NSW, and Canberra;

two items which give some indication of the strength of identification with gay lifestyle: own sexual identity, and attributed sexual identity;

the three scales of gay community attachment: Sexual Engagement (SXE), Social Engagement (SCE) and Gay Community Involvement (GCI);

Table 8.4. Means and Standard Deviations for Knowledge of 'Safe' Sex (KSS) and 'Unsafe' Sex (KUS) Scales for Locale and ANOVA Results

		Inner Sydney	Northern suburbs	Outer Sydney	Extra-metropolitan	Canberra
KSS	Mean:	7.42	6.40	6.75	5.90	8.50
	SD:	3.37	3.09	3.36	2.46	3.39
	N	304	43	63	81	42

$$F_{(4,528)} = 6.18, \ p < 0.0001$$

		Inner Sydney	Northern suburbs	Outer Sydney	Extra-metropolitan	Canberra
KUS	Mean:	6.67	6.98	6.41	7.26	5.69
	SD:	2.19	2.22	2.42	2.07	2.24
	N	304	43	63	81	42

$$F_{(4,528)} = 3.94, \ p < 0.004$$

Source: Kippax *et al.* (1990).

two measures of access to information about HIV transmission: a measure of extent of awareness of exposure to pamphlets and other gay literature — 'pamphlet awareness' (PA), and a measure of active seeking out of information about HIV and safe sex.

Analyses were carried out to assess the impact of these context variables on KSS and KUS scores. Locale was significantly related to both knowledge scales (locale was assessed by comparing Inner Sydney suburbs with the other four). Table 8.4 shows the mean scores on KSS and KUS for each locale.

Locale was the only context variable which was significantly related to scores on KUS. Men who live outside the metropolitan area of Sydney, with the exception of those who live in Canberra, were more likely to be accurate with regard to 'unsafe' practices and/or err on the side of caution and were more likely to assess practices as 'small risk' or 'nor at all safe' than men who live in Inner Sydney. On the other hand, men who live in Canberra or in the Inner Sydney suburbs were more likely to rate practices classified as 'not at all safe' as 'safe' or 'small risk' and hence got low scores on KUS.

Knowledge scores were unrelated to sexual identity and to gay community attachment scores, although scores on KSS, but not scores on KUS, were significantly related to membership of gay organizations ($F_{1,524} = 4.27$, $p < 0.03$). Scores on KSS, unlike scores on KUS, were also significantly related to pamphlet awareness (PA) ($r = 0.118$, $p < 0.0003$) as well as locale. Since these context measures were correlated with one another, a multiple regression analysis was carried out to investigate the extent to which the context variables overlapped in

Table 8.5. *Multiple Regression: Reduced Model for Knowledge of 'Safe' Sex (KSS) Scale*

Predictor variable	r^2 % variance fitted first	Raw regression coefficient	t	p	% variance fitted last
Education	0.35	0.093	0.768	0.443	0.1
Locale[a]	4.47				3.7
Northern suburbs		−0.942	−1.788	0.074	
Outer Sydney		−0.495	−1.093	0.275	
Extra-metropolitan		−1.290	−3.041	0.002	
Canberra		1.215	2.215	0.027	
Pamphlet awareness	1.39	0.153	2.197	0.028	0.9

$R^2 = 5.8\%$ MSE = 10.33 Error df = 519
Significance of regression: $F_{(6,519)} = 5.3$, $p < 0.0005$

Note: a Comparison of each of these locales with inner city.
Source: Kippax *et al*. (1990).

contributing to the scores on KSS. The overall regression was significant ($F_{10,523} = 3.39$, $p < 0.0005$), with $R^2 = 6.2$ per cent. A reduced model, including education, accounted for 5.8 per cent of the variance. Details of this reduced model are shown in Table 8.5.

The importance of pamphlet awareness is highlighted in the investigation of the relationship between attachment to gay community measures (SXE, SCE and GCI), KSS scores with PA scores. A significant amount of variance in KSS scores was accounted for by PA over and above attachment to gay community. The reverse, however, was not true. This finding suggested that attachment to gay community, particularly membership of gay organizations, affects scores on KSS by providing access to safe sex materials, including posters and pamphlets. This relationship held even after the contribution of locale was taken into account. The reduced model, therefore, included only education, locale and pamphlet awareness.

Table 8.6. *Correlations of Gay Community and Knowledge Scales*

Gay Community Attachment	Knowledge scales				
	KSS	KUS	KSP	GI	PA
GCI	0.08	0.03	0.16***	−0.12**	0.48***
SCE	0.08	−0.02	0.16***	−0.08	0.31***
SXE	−0.04	0.03	−0.02	0.01	0.14**
GID	0.03	0.08	0.18***	−0.12**	0.23***

Notes: ** $p < 0.00$ *** $p < 0.001$
Source: SAPA Monograph Report No. 7.

Table 8.7. Sources of Information about AIDS and Safe Sex

Source	First mentioned source	
	AIDS	Safe Sex
	Percentage of respondents (n = 535)	
Mainstream press	47.1	6.5
Gay press	24.5	45.8
Friends	19.8	23.2
Gay organizations	0.6	15.1
Doctors/clinics	2.6	5.2
Other/don't know	5.4	4.2

Source: Kippax *et al.* (1990).

In summary, the analyses indicated the importance of locale and gay community, at least with regard to knowledge of 'safe' sex. Men who lived in Inner Sydney and Canberra, both centres of gay communities where access to gay literature on 'safe' sex is readily available, were more likely to know what is 'safe' and/or when in doubt assessed a practice as 'safe'. Knowledge of 'unsafe' sex, on the other hand, was unrelated to attachment to gay community, although it was related to locale: the more distant men were from centres of gay community, the more likely they were to know what was 'unsafe' and/or when in doubt assessed a practice as 'unsafe'. It appears that these extra-metropolitan men were more likely to rely on the mainstream media for their information about HIV transmission.

That attachment to gay lifestyle is important for the amount of information about 'safe' sex and the accuracy of that knowledge was also indicated by the number of men who cited the gay press, their friends and gay organizations as the main source of information about AIDS and safe sex (see Table 8.7).

As might be expected, the press, both mainstream and gay, plays an important role in informing our sample about AIDS and HIV, but it is the gay community — gay press, friends, gay organizations — which was most often cited (by 84.1 per cent of the respondents) as the main sources of information about 'safe' sex. Men had learnt about AIDS from the mainstream media and that certain practices are dangerous with respect to HIV transmission. They had learnt what they could do and how to do it safely from their own communities. The HIV-related information had not only been positioned differently by these two sources, but the sources, in part, had provided different contexts in which the information was received and transformed.

Locale is not simply a post code; some men choose to live in certain areas because of their association with gay community life. Men's immediate social context appears to be extremely important with respect to availability of information and the way such information is processed and interpreted. If 'well informed' is taken to mean knowledge of 'safe' sex, then, as DiClemente, Zorn and Temoshok (1987) found, people living close to the AIDS epicentre were the most well informed. But in the SAPA study those living close to the epicentre were not the only ones well informed with respect to 'safe' sex. Men who lived in Canberra, a relatively long way from the epicentre, were as well, if not better, informed (Kippax *et al.*, 1990). Knowledge is not simply a function of closeness to the epidemic; attachment to gay community is also important. As Fisher (1988) noted: degree of involvement in gay community social networks figures importantly in exposure to normative and informational social influence with regard to behaviours consistent with AIDS prevention.

Two Patterns of Knowledge

These findings explain, in large part, the curious finding of a negative correlation between knowledge of 'safe' sexual practices and knowledge of 'unsafe' practices. Men not only made their judgments of safety in terms of information available to them at the time; some of them also overestimated or underestimated the safety of sexual practices. These judgments were in turn linked to locale, attachment to gay community and sexual practice.

With regard to sexual practice and its role in knowledge, our analysis of knowledge of 'safe' and 'unsafe' sexual practices also revealed a very consistent relationship between engagement in a particular sexual activity and a tendency to judge that activity as safe (Kippax *et al.*, 1990). It was not possible to tell from the data whether the men in the study thought a particular practice was safe because they engaged in it or vice versa. Psychological studies suggest that if there is any influence of one on the other, it is probably bidirectional (Calder and Ross, 1973).

Gay and bisexual men in the sample who were geographically isolated from or unattached to gay community were less likely to know which sexual practices they could enjoy without risk; their knowledge of 'safe' sexual practices, as defined by the AIDS Council of NSW in 1987, was not as accurate as that of men who lived in Canberra or inner Sydney. These men, in the latter category, were also more likely to engage in a wide range of sexual practice.

Conclusions

Our findings indicated that knowledge was not acquired in a simple fashion. Its reception is dependent upon the context in which the message is sent and received. The gay media have been extremely important. The men in this study had made use of the gay media to inform themselves about HIV transmission and the safety of a number of sexual practices. The two sources of information, the mainstream and the gay media, had had a differential impact. Gay and bisexual men need more information about sexual practices other than anal inter-course, particularly those men who are isolated from gay community. The focus of this information should be on what is safe rather than what is risky; on what men who have sex with men can do and how to do it safely.

The findings also indicated that men who are isolated from gay community are more cautious with regard to what they consider 'safe' sexual practice. This may at first sight seem a positive outcome of the mainstream media, but abstaining from a wide range of sexual prac-tices, even practices the health authorities consider safe, may be counterproductive. Such abstinence may be difficult to sustain over time. As discussed in Chapter 7, changes in sexual practice are related to knowledge of 'safe' and 'unsafe' sex. Men who are isolated from gay community and who have relatively little knowledge of what sexual practices they may engage in safely are more likely than men not so isolated to change the nature of their sexual relationships rather than adopt safe sexual practice. Relationship changes may not prevent HIV transmission.

The most successful education campaigns are those which can be integrated with existing community mores and meanings. Knowledge is not absorbed in a passive way; men transform information in ways that make it intelligible to themselves and their sexual partners. Gay community, through its press and education campaigns, has produced a climate of safe sexual practice. In 1992 in Sydney and Canberra gay community attached men have to explain why no condoms, not argue for their use.

Chapter 9

Gay Community Attachment

Attachment to gay community takes many forms. Three measures of attachment have been identified and used in the analysis of the SAPA data: sexual engagement, social engagement and gay community involvement. In this chapter we describe these three forms of gay community attachment, examine the relationships between them and other social factors, such as place of residence and closeness to the epicentre of the HIV epidemic. As described in Chapters 7 and 8, attachment to gay community has played a significant role in HIV prevention. We investigate the nature of this role in this Chapter.

In Western countries, where gay men were among the first to suffer from infection by the human immunodeficiency virus, gay communities took the lead in HIV prevention campaigns. For example, North American gay communities were among the first to suggest condoms to prevent the transmission of HIV in anal intercourse. In Australia gay communities developed some of the most successful initiatives in Australian AIDS education. Dowsett (1989a, 1989b) has documented the importance of the gay community in Sydney as a source of information and educational material about HIV and 'safe sex', and we review much of this material in Chapter 2. In the United Kingdom, too, gay communities have taken a major role (see Fitzpatrick, Boulton and Hart, 1989; Watney, 1990).

Among health educators there is a firm commitment to the importance of gay communities in HIV prevention. In a discussion of comprehensive risk reduction strategies for adolescents, DiClemente, Boyer and Mills (1987) point to the need for culturally relevant and sensitive educational material. Educational messages most likely to succeed are those which speak the language of the particular audience to which the messages are directed. Graham and Cates (1987) discuss the importance of initiatives taken by the leaders of the gay community in establishing an AIDS task force in Indiana; and Williams (1986) describes the development of a strategy to encourage members of at-risk populations to assume leadership roles in education efforts to reduce HIV transmission.

At the time of the SAPA study few studies of sexual behaviour change found any evidence of a consistent relationship between gay community attachment and change in sexual behaviour in response to HIV. For example, in the United States, Emmons *et al.* (1986) report that although knowledge of HIV transmission was related to reported behaviour change, social norms were related only to a certain type of behaviour change, namely that concerning the number or type of one's sexual partners.

Given the beliefs of health educators and their commitment to community education programs, these research results are puzzling. Perhaps the reason for not finding the expected relationship between gay community and behaviour change lies in the complexity of the meaning of gay community, the individualistic bias of the health belief models (as noted in Chapter 8) and their subsequent difficulty in adequately capturing that complexity in any survey measure. Certainly, the assessment of the impact of attachment to gay community on the up-take of information or behaviour change is complicated by the fact that there is usually considerable overlap between attachment to gay community and the AIDS epicentre. DiClemente, Zorn and Temoshok (1987) noted, in their comparison of surveys conducted in the United States of America, that proximity to an AIDS epicentre has great saliency with respect to knowledge and attitudes about HIV/AIDS.

Gay men living in the Castro Street area in San Francisco and around Oxford Street in Sydney, both areas with a large gay population, are more likely to have an attachment to gay culture and community as well as a high degree of contact with the epidemic. Men who live in these areas are very likely to have had friends who have died of AIDS and to know others who are infected with HIV. Any change of sexual behaviour is likely to be related to all three variables: attachment to gay community, place of residence and contact with the epidemic.

A sense of gay community is constituted in practices, both sexual and social. It is produced and has been transformed over time in gay bars and discos, at gay political meetings and rallies, in 'beats' (places such as parks or public toilets where men may meet other men for sex), in homes and social gatherings; it is constructed in political and social activity and in sexual practice. As Altman (1979, 1982) among others has noted, the HIV epidemic has reinforced an already strong sense of community among gay men.

At the same time gay identity, identification of self as gay, has been transformed. It, too, is constructed in practice, both social and sexual, as well as in sexual preferences. As Weeks (1987: 31) said of gay identity: 'For many in the modern world — especially the sexually marginal — it is an absolutely fundamental concept, offering a sense of personal unity, social location, and even at times a political commitment.'

The analysis we undertook focused on the development of gay identity and gay community scales which captured the complexity noted above. We also examined the relationship of these measures to the social descriptor variables and to those variables we called milieu variables, place of residence and the closeness to the epidemic measures.

Measures of Gay Identity and Attachment to Gay Community

Over sixty questions in the questionnaire concerned sexual identity, various forms of attachment to gay community and engagement in and identification with gay life. There were a number of questions about membership of gay organizations; further questions dealt with the places and venues where respondents sought contact of a social and sexual kind; others dealt with whether the respondents patronized gay businesses, read gay newspapers and went to gay doctors.

The responses to all these items were intercorrelated and factor analyzed. These analyses were interrogated with a view to constructing a number of gay identity and gay community scales. The majority of men surveyed considered themselves gay (89 per cent). Of the remainder who did not identify as gay, 7 per cent considered themselves bisexual, 1 per cent identified as heterosexual, while the rest were unsure. Well over half the men (65 per cent) believed that others knew of their gay identity, while 17 per cent believed that others considered they were heterosexual and 6 per cent believed that others knew they were bisexual. The remaining 12 per cent did not know what others thought.

Although no scale was found that gave a direct measure of gay identity, we were able to construct a reliable scale, the Gay Identity Disclosure Scale (see Table 9.1). As the name implies, this scale (GID) measured the degree to which men had disclosed their sexual identity to others (parents, friends, workmates, neighbours). Most men in our sample had disclosed their sexual identity to someone, friends and workmates being the most likely; and most men had disclosed to around four categories of persons (mean scale score was 4.2).

Table 9.1. *Gay Identity Disclosure (GID) Scale*

Item	Item mean	Item-total correlation
1 Mother	0.63	0.58
2 Father	0.49	0.55
3 Other relative	0.66	0.46
4 Straight friends	0.90	0.31
5 Workmates	0.75	0.41
6 Neighbours	0.39	0.34
7 Other people	0.36	0.34
	Cronbach's alpha: 0.72	

Source: Kippax *et al.* (1992).

No single factor of gay community attachment emerged. The exploratory factor analyses suggested the existence of at least three scales. Attachment is not unitary and takes various forms. We named these three scales Gay Community Involvement (GCI), Social Engagement in Gay Community (SCE) and Sexual Engagement in Gay Community (SXE).

In essence, the Gay Community Involvement scale measures the degree of men's 'immersion' in modern gay culture and politics. The scale, a reliable one, has twenty-one items and the item-total correlations are shown in Table 9.2. The scores ranged from 20 to 46 and were normally distributed around the mean scale score of 32.6 with a standard deviation of 5.2. Someone with a high score on this scale would be likely to read gay newspapers, patronize gay shops and businesses, go to a gay-identified doctor, attend gay functions (sporting, political, social) and be a member of gay organizations, social, political and AIDS-related.

Another ten items formed a scale which we identified as a measure of social engagement in gay community, the Social Engagement scale (SCE). The items and the item-total correlations are shown in Table 9.3. The scores ranged from 9 to 23, the mean scale score was 19.0, and the standard deviation was 2.5. The scores on this scale were skewed with the majority of men scoring between 20 and 23; that is, most men had a degree of social contact with other gay and bisexual men. Men with relatively high scores on this scale were likely to have gay male friends. They were also likely to spend much of their free time with gay men, and much of their social contact took place in gay bars, discos as well as private parties and meetings. These men's attachment was lived out in terms of a social engagement with gay community.

A third scale, which we called the Sexual Engagement scale (SXE), was made up of nineteen items which measure the number of casual

Table 9.2. Gay Community Involvement (GCI) Scale

Item		Item mean	Item-total correlation
1	Identifies with gay community (g.c.)	2.73	0.36
2	Goes to gay-identified doctor	2.10	0.32
3	Reads gay newspapers	2.46	0.36
4	Goes to g.c. sporting functions	1.27	0.30
5	Goes to g.c. political functions	1.24	0.41
6	Goes to g.c. social group functions	1.59	0.44
7	Goes to g.c. religious functions	1.13	0.23
8	Goes to g.c. counselling groups	1.24	0.39
9	Goes to g.c. AIDS-related groups	1.35	0.43
10	Goes to g.c. university/college groups	1.10	0.16
11	Member of g.c. organizations	1.67	0.59
12	Member of g.c. sporting group	1.15	0.29
13	Member of g.c. political group	1.26	0.43
14	Member of g.c. social group	1.48	0.48
15	Member of g.c. religious group	1.13	0.27
16	Member of g.c. counselling group	1.26	0.46
17	Member of g.c. AIDS-related group	1.32	0.50
18	Member of g.c. university/college group	1.15	0.26
19	Patronizes gay shops and businesses	1.87	0.40
20	Goes to gay films/theatre	2.12	0.43
21	Reads books with gay themes	1.96	0.43
	Cronbach's alpha: 0.81		

Source: Kippax *et al.* (1992).

Table 9.3. Social Engagement (SCE) Scale

Item		Item mean	Item-total correlation
1	Spends free time with gay friends	3.50	0.50
2	Friends are gay men	1.58	0.45
3	Goes out with gay friends (g.f.)	1.96	0.40
4	Goes out with g.f. to bars	1.79	0.40
5	Goes out with g.f. to theatre/films	1.89	0.41
6	Goes out with g.f. to discos/dances	1.72	0.44
7	Goes out with g.f. to private parties	1.89	0.47
8	Goes out with g.f. to bookshops	1.26	0.21
9	Goes out with g.f. to pool/beach	1.75	0.38
10	Goes out with g.f. to meetings	1.71	0.28
	Cronbach's alpha: 0.71		

Source: Kippax *et al.* (1992).

partners and the frequency of casual sex, as well as men's use of sex venues such as saunas and beats to find partners, both social and sexual. In essence, this scale captures men's sexual engagement with gay community. The items and the item-total correlations are shown in Table 9.4.

The scores on this scale ranged from 17 to 40 with a mean scale score of 25.2 and a standard deviation of 4.5. The distribution was

Table 9.4. *Sexual Engagement (SXE) Scale*

Item		Item mean	Item-total correlation
1	Number of casual partners in last six months	1.80	0.62
2	Frequency of casual sex	0.85	0.59
3	Uses gay video pornography	1.86	0.19
4	Seeks sexual partners at bars	1.66	0.43
5	Seeks sexual partners at saunas	1.39	0.51
6	Seeks sexual partners at discos	1.59	0.38
7	Seeks sexual partners at parties	1.68	0.35
8	Seeks sexual partners at beats	1.37	0.51
9	Seeks sexual partners at bookshops	1.13	0.34
10	Seeks sexual partners at sex cinema	1.04	0.28
11	Seeks male prostitutes	1.04	0.22
12	Seeks sexual partners at gym	1.16	0.21
13	Seeks sexual partners at pool/beach	1.43	0.37
14	Seeks social contact at saunas	1.19	0.39
15	Seeks social contact at beats	1.12	0.29
16	Seeks social contact at sex cinema	1.03	0.17
17	Seeks social contact at wall*	1.02	0.14
18	Uses venues for sex with casual partner	1.69	0.63
19	Uses venues for sex with regular partner	1.15	0.21
	Cronbach's alpha: 0.79		

Note: * A place for meeting young male prostitutes.
Source: Kippax *et al.* (1992).

slightly negatively skewed: most men had some degree of sexual engagement in gay community, but some, approximately 20 per cent, had little sexual engagement in gay community as measured by this scale.

Thus the analysis revealed three forms of attachment to gay community, cultural/political, social and sexual, and a measure of public commitment as captured by the Gay Identity Disclosure scale. All four measures were intercorrelated. Although the high correlation between the GCI and SCE scales suggested the possibility of a single scale, the content of the two sets of items is sufficiently different to keep them separate (see Table 9.5). The relatively small correlations between the Sexual Engagement scale and the other two gay community attachment scales indicated that men who engage in casual sex and seek sexual partners in a variety of venues are not necessarily socially or culturally/politically involved in gay community.

There were strong positive correlations between the Gay Identity Disclosure scale and both the Gay Community Involvement and Social Engagement scales, but no relationship between it and the Sexual Engagement scale was found. These data indicated a stronger public commitment to gay community among the men whose attachment is either cultural/political or social as opposed to sexual. Also indicated is

Table 9.5. Relationship between Gay Identity Disclosure and Community Attachment Scales

| | Correlations between the scales | | | |
	Gay Identity Disclosure	Gay Community Involvement	Social Engagement	Sexual Engagement
GID	1.00	0.34*	0.25*	0.05
GCI		1.00	0.48*	0.17*
SCE			1.00	0.22*
SXE				1.00

Note: * p < 0.001
Source: Kippax *et al.* (1992).

that some men who are sexually engaged with other men have kept this aspect of their life hidden from their family, friends and social networks. In gay community parlance these men might be described as being 'in the closet'. This does not necessarily mean that these men were uncomfortable about their gay identity or sexual preference. Men who are sexually engaged in gay community but who have told few others of their sexual interest may be perfectly at home with their sexuality, but deem it unnecessary or perhaps unsafe to tell others. Indeed, in this sample of men with 89 per cent describing themselves as gay, adjustment to any personal acceptance of sexual preference would not appear a problem.

Self-attributed gay identity and other-attributed gay identity were also significantly related to the Gay Community Involvement scale (F = 10.19, p < 0.0015; F = 17.54, p < 0.0000) and the Social Engagement scale (F = 27.1, p < 0.0000; F = 19.42, p < 0.0000). In both cases attribution of 'gay' identity, by self or other, was positively related to involvement in and social engagement with gay community. Also, as one might expect, men who identified as 'gay' were more likely to have disclosed their sexual orientation to others (F = 6.4, p < 0.01). Men who identify as gay are active in gay community life; this attachment, in turn, confirms men's identity as gay.

Sexual engagement was not associated with self- or other-attributed identity (F = 1.45, NS; F = 2.30, NS). This could mean that sexual identity is not constituted in sexual engagement in gay community and/or that sexual engagement alone has little to do with seeing oneself or being seen by others as gay. The data indicated that men with low scores on the GCI and SCE scales were relatively less likely to identify as gay whatever the strength or diversity of their sexual engagement.

In general, a strong sense of commitment to gay identity, both public and personal, appeared to be related to social engagement in and cultural/political involvement in gay life. Gay community attachment also manifested itself in the form of a sexual engagement. This type of attachment was only marginally related to either cultural/political involvement or social engagement in gay community and was independent of self- or other-attributed 'gay' identity as well as disclosure of that identity.

Social Descriptor Variables in Relation to Gay Community

Further analysis revealed that these four scales were related to a number of descriptor variables such as age, education and, very importantly, place of residence (see Table 9.6). While men from all social backgrounds and classes participated in the social and sexual offerings of gay community life, cultural and political involvement was limited to middle-class men. The Gay Community Involvement scale was the only scale to show significant and positive relationships with a number of social descriptor variables — education, occupational status and income. It may be that these middle-class men were and continue to be a substantial part of the gay liberation movement.

Age was related to the two engagement scales. There was more active sexual engagement in gay community among men aged 30 years and older and less social engagement among men aged 39 and over. There was a slight tendency among the young to favour a social rather than a sexual engagement in gay community life, perhaps as one result of the impact of HIV.

These data confirmed our initial interpretation: that there are three forms of gay community attachment captured by our data. This does not mean that there are three types of gay man. Rather, the data indicated that there are men whose attachment to gay community is expressed in all three ways outlined below, others for whom attachment is constituted in only one or two of these forms and others for whom any form of attachment is minimal.

These three forms may be characterized in the following ways: the first as measured on the GCI Scale is primarily a cultural and political involvement. Men with a strong gay community involvement are likely to be middle-class professional men who are confident in their identity and have disclosed it to many — their relatives, friends, workmates and neighbours.

Table 9.6. Gay Community Attachment and Identity Disclosure Scale Mean Scores on Social Descriptor Variables

Mean scale scores	GCI	SCE	SXE	GID
Age:				
<19	31.27	19.05	24.32	3.45
20–29	32.25	19.38	24.35	4.18
30–39	32.86	19.13	26.09	4.46
40–49	32.96	18.38	25.25	3.78
50+	33.06	17.96	24.96	3.50
	NS	***	***	*
National origin:	NS	NS	NS	NS
Religion:				
Agnostic	33.30	19.12	24.95	4.52
Protestant	32.35	19.19	25.39	3.98
Catholic	32.01	18.78	25.24	3.59
Other	31.16	18.77	25.42	4.04
	*	NS	NS	***
Education:				
Up to Year 11	30.99	18.80	25.60	3.86
Years 11 and 12	32.51	19.26	25.28	4.21
Post-secondary	31.70	18.94	25.01	4.35
Higher education	33.75	19.07	24.95	4.30
	***	NS	NS	NS
Occupation:				
Managerial/Professional	33.38	19.18	25.31	4.38
Paraprofessional	32.57	19.05	24.80	3.97
Sales/Unskilled	31.56	18.95	26.22	4.05
	*	NS	NS	NS
Income:				
<12,000	31.27	18.70	24.55	4.32
12,001–18,000	32.76	19.22	25.16	4.09
18,001–26,000	33.08	19.30	25.40	4.18
26,001+	33.04	19.00	25.47	4.20
	*	NS	NS	NS
Labour force status:	NS	NS	NS	NS

Notes: * $p < 0.05$ ** $p < 0.01$ *** $p < 0.005$
Levels of significance are for ANOVAS.
Source: Kippax et al. (1992).

The second takes the form of a social engagement, as measured by the SCE scale. Those whose attachment is social are younger but in terms of class are a far more heterogeneous group than those with a cultural and political involvement. Like the men with a cultural and political involvement, these socially attached men identify as gay and are likely to disclose their identity to others. Their gay identity is constituted in their friendships and their leisure pursuits, but not necessarily in their membership of gay organizations.

The third form of attachment is characterized by sexual engagement as measured by the SXE scale. They are a heterogeneous group of men, although more likely to be older than those who have a social engagement with gay culture. Although they are less likely than men with a cultural and political involvement or social engagement in gay community to have disclosed their sexual preferences to others, they are just as likely to identify themselves and be identified by others as gay, or bisexual or heterosexual. It is as though their identity is constituted in sexual rather than social or cultural/political practices, and, for many, their sexual practices are separate from the rest of their lives.

Gay Community, Locale and Contact with HIV

Place of residence is an important concept with regard to gay community and HIV transmission. Oxford Street and the inner-city suburbs are the suburbs in which many gay men choose to live. One hundred and twenty-one men, 22.6 per cent of the sample, had moved to Sydney in the last five years, and 85 per cent of these men had moved to the inner-Sydney suburbs. These areas house many of the gay bars, discos, saunas, businesses and meeting places. As noted in Chapter 7, a variable we called 'Locale' was created to assess place of residence. The five locales are Inner Sydney, which takes in Oxford Street, the eastern suburbs of Sydney and the inner city and is the cosmopolitan area of Sydney housing many of its restaurants and bars, cinemas and theatres, discos and nightclubs, as well as the public focus of much gay activity in Sydney; Northern suburbs which house the professional upper-middle class; Outer Sydney, which takes in the southern, western, and south-western suburbs, which are, in the main, the suburbs of the working and lower-middle classes; Extra-metropolitan New South Wales including its industrial cities and country towns; and Canberra which, as the seat of the Australian federal government, is populated by public servants, well educated professional men and women.

Place of residence or locale is important because of claims that changes in sexual practice have occurred *because* of gay men's contact with the epidemic. The epicentre of HIV/AIDS is identified with the Oxford Street and inner-Sydney area. Men who live in this area are likely to have had more contact with the epidemic, as well as more

Table 9.7. *Mean Gay Community and Contact with the Epidemic Scores by Locale*

Mean scale scores	GCI	SCE	SXE	GID	CE
Locale					
Inner Sydney	33.42	19.53	25.59	4.53	1.75
Northern Suburbs	32.41	18.81	25.22	4.09	1.19
Outer Sydney	31.05	18.55	24.98	3.22	0.91
Extra-metropolitan NSW	30.19	18.15	24.19	4.19	1.06
Canberra	33.03	19.15	24.00	3.38	0.75
	***	***	NS	***	***

Notes: *** $p < 0.001$
Levels of significance are for ANOVAs.
Source: Kippax *et al.* (1992).

contact with gay community responses to HIV/AIDS, than men who live in the outer suburbs and outside Sydney. A variable to assess degree of contact with the epidemic, CE, was developed from three items: knowing anyone with AIDS, caring or nursing people with AIDS, and knowing anyone who has died of AIDS (see Connell *et al.*, 1989). The relationship between contact with the epidemic and men's test status (untested, negative, positive) and gay community attachment was also examined.

Locale was significantly associated with a cultural/political involvement and social engagement in gay community as well as disclosure of gay identity. It was also significantly related to contact with the epidemic (see Table 9.7).

While men in Inner Sydney had the strongest attachments to gay community and men in Outer Sydney and in Extra-metropolitan NSW were least likely to be socially engaged or involved in gay community, men in all locales had some form of attachment to gay community. That is, although the Inner Sydney locale is better supplied with bars, discos and saunas, all locales are able to offer meeting places for social, cultural/political and sexual contact. The most striking aspect of Table 9.7 is that, unlike the other gay community attachment measures, the SXE scale is unrelated to locale. Men's sexual engagement with gay community is unrelated to place of residence.

Contact with the Epidemic was, as predicted, greatest for those men who live in Inner Sydney, and proportionally more of these Inner Sydney men had been tested than in any other locale (73.4 per cent compared with 51.8 per cent in Extra-metropolitan NSW and 55.5 per cent in Outer Sydney). Test status was also significantly related to measures of gay community attachment and gay identity disclosure (see Table 9.8). Those men with the strongest attachment to gay com-

Table 9.8. Mean Gay Community and Contact with the Epidemic Scores by Test Status

Mean scale scores					
	GCI	SCE	SXE	GID	CE
Test status					
Untested	31.1	18.5	24.2	3.7	1.2
Test-negative	33.0	19.2	25.4	4.4	1.5
Test-positive	34.0	19.6	26.5	4.5	1.8
	***	***	***	***	***

Notes: *** $p < 0.001$
　　　Levels of significance are for ANOVAs.
Source: Kippax *et al.* (1992).

munity and those who were more likely to have disclosed their identity were more likely to have been tested than not. Note, however, that the outcome of the test was unrelated to these gay community measures.

Summary of Scales and Relationship with Other Measures

Gay community attachment was far more closely related to locale and contact with the epidemic than to the social descriptor variables discussed above. The social descriptors were, with the exception of the class-related variables, unrelated to gay community, whereas locale, contact with the epidemic and test status (tested versus untested) were very closely related to gay community measures. Respondents who lived in Inner Sydney embraced gay life. Of these, men who were well educated were likely to have a strong sense of gay community involvement, while the young were likely to have a social engagement with gay community. Men who live in Inner Sydney were also likely to have disclosed their identity to most others; they appeared confident in their gay identity. These men were also the men with the greatest contact with the epidemic.

Men who live in other locales, however, were also attached to gay community, but in different ways. Some were culturally and politically involved and others were socially engaged. Locale may limit the *ways* in which these forms of attachment are lived, but it does not appear to limit the attachment itself. Sexual engagement is, however, unaffected by locale: it was independent of locale and most of the social descriptors.

Table 9.9. *Mean Gay Community and Contact with the Epidemic Scores by Relationship Status*

Mean scale scores	GCI	SCE	SXE	GID
Relationship status				
No relationship	33.2	19.4	23.0	4.4
Monogamous	32.1	19.2	21.0	4.1
Regular plus[a]	33.3	19.4	26.6	4.7
Several relationships	33.9	19.6	27.7	4.3
Casual only	31.7	19.1	27.0	3.7
	*	**	***	***

Notes: * $p < 0.05$ ** $p < 0.01$ *** $p < 0.005$
   a Regular partner plus casual sexual relations for either or both partners.
   Levels of significance are for ANOVAs.
Source: Kippax et al. (1992).

Gay Community Attachment and Sexual Practice

The above picture of gay community attachment is rounded out by an examination of the relationship between attachment and sexual practice. Although there were no significant relationships between locale and nature of sexual relationships, all three gay community attachment scales and the gay identity disclosure measures are significantly related to relationship status (see Table 9.9). Men in monogamous relationships and those with only casual partners had the weakest attachment to gay community. Although those with only casual partners had a strong sexual engagement in gay community, their cultural/political involvement and social engagement was weak. These men were also the least likely to tell others of their homosexual interest. Men in regular relationships in which either they or their partners also had casual sex were most strongly attached to gay community.

Similarly for sexual practice: although locale had no impact on sexual practice, attachment to gay community, particularly social and sexual engagement, was significantly related to sexual practice. As noted in Chapter 7, the stronger the engagement in gay community, the more varied the sexual practice. It is important to note, however, that although sexual practice was more varied for men with strong social and political involvement in gay community, men with weak attachment to gay community as measured on GCI and SCE were more likely to engage in dangerous practice with casual partners, as defined in Chapter 6. On the other hand, men who had a strong sexual engagement in gay community were more likely to have a more varied sexual practice and to engage in dangerous practice with casual partners.

Sophistication in sexual relationships and sexual practice is associated with gay community attachment. Sex venues perhaps play a role here, and social engagement in gay community appears to offer scope for sexual encounters. The older men in the sample were more likely to use the sex venues; the younger men relied on the social networks. Locale, however, was not important. If there are no saunas, discos or backroom bars, informal venues and meeting places, such as beats, take their place. These informal venues also often provide anonymity and privacy.

Thus the three forms of gay community attachment identified and discussed earlier in this chapter were closely related to locale and contact with the epidemic. This was especially true for the forms of gay community attachment captured by the Gay Community Involvement scale and the Social Engagement scale. These two forms of attachment are closely linked to each other and to gay identity disclosure; they express a social and cultural/political commitment to living a gay life. For younger gay men, gay life is more likely to be social than cultural/political; unlike their older counterparts, their introduction to gay community was probably forged after gay liberation began to have an impact on the lives of homosexual men. It is of interest to note, however, that the men who live in the Extra-metropolitan NSW and the Inner Sydney locales were more likely to have disclosed their identity to others.

The Inner Sydney, Northern suburbs and Canberra locales offer a greater range of forms of attachment to gay community. Locale, however, does not limit sexual expression. Attachment to gay community is also associated with a greater variety of expression of sexuality. Being gay takes many forms — social, sexual, cultural/political — and is lived out in a variety of ways, publicly and privately, in different places.

Gay Community and Changing Sexual Practice

We summarized the relationship between gay community attachment and changes to sexual practice in Chapter 7. The best predictors of the adoption of safe sexual practice were: sexual and social engagement in gay community — the greater the engagement, the greater the adoption of safe sex; educational status — those with more years of education were more likely to have changed their sexual practices in the direction of safe sex; knowledge of unsafe sexual practices — an accurate knowledge of 'unsafe' sexual practices contributed to the adoption of 'safe' sexual practices; and locale — men who lived in Extra-metropolitan NSW changed least when compared with men from Inner Sydney. Contact with the epidemic was not important once gay community attachment and locale variables were taken into account. A detailed statistical examination is found in Crawford, Kippax and Dowsett (1990).

The best predictors of relationship change were a lack of knowledge of 'safe' sexual practices, a lack of education, and a minimal sexual engagement in gay community. Men who lived in Extra-metropolitan NSW and in the Northern suburbs of Sydney compared with those in the Inner Sydney suburbs were most likely to change their relationships.

These findings point to the importance of informed social support. The importance of gay community is obvious. Men who have little gay community attachment, have little knowledge of 'safe' sexual practice, and rely on mainstream media are more likely to change the form of their relationships, to move towards monogamy and celibacy and to reduce the number of their casual partners, in response to HIV. Men in contact with others, via attachments to gay community, sexual and social, are most likely to have changed their sexual practice. They have the informed social support necessary to modify their behaviour. Men who are isolated from others like themselves and are unattached to gay community in any form are those least likely to change. Some of these 'unattached' men have changed because of their contact with the epidemic; others have not. In order to protect themselves, some of them appear to have changed the nature of their sexual relationships. Those most likely to have made these moves are those who live away from the public centres of gay community. Gay community, especially, in its social, cultural and political forms, provides gay men with a supportive environment that enables the negotiation of safe sex. The cultural backdrop in which men find partners and negotiate sex has changed.

This raises a question about the continued coyness and lack of clarity with respect to male-to-male sex and HIV transmission in Australian national AIDS education campaigns. Gay community education efforts work; but they only reach so far beyond the local gay communities, and they rely on some form of attachment to gay community. Either gay community education needs to be resourced sufficiently and charged with the responsibility of reaching out far beyond its current focus or mainstream education is going to have to bite the bullet and become more explicit and determined to reach all men who have sex with men.

Chapter 10

Bisexuality: Identity and Practice

In the debate about the spread of HIV and AIDS, 'bisexual' men are described as a possible bridge via which the epidemic will cross over from the gay to the general (assumed heterosexual) population (for example, Anderson and May, 1992). The issue of 'bisexuality' is a very complex one and there are many different ways in which bisexuality can be understood. It is too simplistic to believe that there is a single bisexual lifestyle.

To assume that all bisexual men practise dangerous forms of sex with their male partners may be inappropriate. In Australia there is little evidence for transmission of HIV from 'bisexual' men to the general population. Heterosexual transmission of AIDS accounts for only 2.5 per cent of the total national AIDS cases (see Chapter 2) — a figure small enough to convince some that AIDS is essentially a problem for gay men only. Even though there has been an increase over time and heterosexual transmission accounted for 5 per cent of HIV infections in 1991, the numbers are quite small. World-wide, however, it is estimated that between 60 and 80 per cent of cases result from heterosexual transmission (Chin, 1991). In both the United States and particularly Great Britain the increase in heterosexual transmission over the past two years has been dramatic, though here too numbers remain relatively small (Anderson and May, 1992).

At the same time as there is discussion about the danger posed to the general population by bisexual men, there is a tendency in literature focusing on the gay community (including some of our own reports) to link 'gay and bisexual', as if clear thinking about the 'bisexual' part of that phrase existed, and therefore that education for and research work on bisexual men had already been carried out. In fact, little is known about bisexual behaviour. Even less is known about who bisexual men are, and the assumption that bisexuality exists as a unitary concept has yet to be tested.

Some conceptual difficulties surround the concept of bisexuality and the question of the relationship between the practice of sex with both male and female partners and the existence of a bisexual 'identity'. Even in our own research we have used the term 'gay and bisexual men' or 'gay/bisexual' as if the words 'gay' and 'bisexual' had the same status, when clearly they do not. Whereas 'gay' is a construct that has been forged out of political, sexual and academic discourse, 'bisexual' is merely a description of a set of sexual practices. The warning of Kinsey (Kinsey, Pomeroy and Martin, 1948) that the term 'a bisexual' was highly problematic still stands.

Many studies of homosexually active men have included explicitly or implicitly men who are bisexually active, but have not separately reported data on the latter group. In this chapter we compare the small group of bisexually active men in our sample with the remainder of the SAPA group. We are aware of the many complex definitional and conceptual issues surrounding the construct of 'bisexuality' (see, for example, Boulton and Coxon, 1991; Crawford *et al.*, 1992), but report here on one aspect only — that of bisexual practice as defined below.

Men Who Have Sex with Both Men and Women in the SAPA Study

The sample of 535 men included many who would be deemed 'bisexual' in one or other sense of the word. Some information about the characteristics of this wider group are given below. However, this chapter concentrates on a group of fifty men who at the time of the survey were 'having sex with men' and who had had sex with a woman during the previous six months. We also examine the ways in which these men differed from the remainder of the men in the sample, their sexual practice, information about HIV, change in sexual practice and gay community attachment. Because of the ways in which we recruited our sample, these men who were having sex with both men and women are likely to be more closely associated with the gay community than are other 'bisexual' men.

There were four questions in the SAPA study relating to the issue of 'bisexuality': sexual identity — 'how do you see yourself'; sexual preference — 'whom do you prefer to have sex with'; a question relating to number of female partners in the previous six months; and a question regarding whether they had ever had sex with a woman. Table 10.1 shows the numbers of men who had had sex with a woman in the previous six months. Response categories for the question about

Table 10.1. *Sex with a Woman in the Past Six Months by Sexual Identity*

Sex with a woman in past six months

	Yes	No	NR/DK	Total	Percentage
Sexual identity					
Gay/camp/homosexual	22	445	8	475	88.8
Bisexual	23	17	0	40	7.5
Other	5	15	0	20	3.7
Total	50	477	8	535	100.0

Note: The fifty men in the 'Yes' column in this table are those labelled 'SMW' in the remainder of this report.

Preferred sex of sexual partners

	Men only	Men and women	NR/DK/None	Total
Sexual identity				
Gay/camp/homosexual	443	27	5	475
Bisexual	11	29	0	40
Other	10	9	1	20
Total	464	65	6	535

Number of female partners ever

	NR/DK	None	1	2–10	11–20	>20	Total
Sexual identity							
Gay/camp/homosexual	11	155	81	188	25	15	475
Bisexual	0	1	3	24	4	8	40
Other	2	1	2	10	2	3	20
Percentage	2.4	29.3	16.1	41.5	5.8	4.8	100.0

Source: SAPA Report No. 8.

sexual identity have been collapsed so that the category 'gay' includes the response 'homosexual' and also terms such as 'camp.'

Most of the 535 men identified themselves as 'gay', 'camp', or 'homosexual', including twenty-two of the men who had had sex with women or had done so within the past six months. Twenty-seven of these self-identified gay men indicated that they preferred to have sex with men and women. There were forty-five men who identified themselves as 'bisexual'; twenty-three of these had had sex with a woman during the previous six months, although twenty-nine expressed a preference for sex with men and women. Five men who identified themselves in some other way had had sex with a woman during the past six months, and fifteen men who identified themselves in some other way had not. Most of the men who had had sex with a woman had had between two and ten female partners. As noted at the end of Table 10.1, the fifty men who had had sex with a woman in the past six months are those who are labelled 'SMW' (Sex with Men and Women) in the remainder of this chapter.

The remaining 485 men in the sample are labelled 'SMO/SIB'; 'SMO' (Sex with Men Only) and 'SIB' (Self-Identified Bisexual). SIB is the label used for the seventeen men who called themselves 'bisexual' but who had not at the time of the survey had sex with a woman within the previous six months. Where we discuss men's experiences of sex with women or issues involving living with or communicating with wife and/or children, the men who self-identified as bisexual but were not currently having sex with women (those labelled SIB) are separated from the men designated as SMO.

Thus for purpose of comparison, we use the following:

SMW: men who were having sex with men and who were also having sex with women (n = 50);

SIB: men who self-identified as bisexual but who at the time of the survey were having sex only with men (n = 17);

SMO: men who self-identified as gay/homosexual/other who at the time of the survey were having sex only with men (n = 468); and

SMO/SIB: SMO plus SIB (n = 485).

The fact that 42.5 per cent of the men who called themselves 'bisexual' had not had sex with a woman in the past six months suggests that these are men who considered themselves bisexual but were living essentially as gay men. They are like the men labelled 'transitional' by Boulton and Coxon (1991). The fifty men who were still having sex with women would satisfy the definition of 'bisexual' as far as most people are concerned, and would represent 'concurrent bisexuality' in Boulton and Coxon's terms. Concurrent bisexuality is most relevant in the context of HIV transmission.

It is noteworthy that only a minority (29 per cent) of the men in the sample had *never* had sex with a woman. Thus, according to many definitions, the majority of men who have sex with men are 'bisexual'. The proportion of these men who have had sex with a woman (69 per cent) agrees very closely with estimates from other populations (Gochros, 1991, quotes a review study by Reinish giving the proportion as 70 per cent).

Table 10.2. Relationship Status of SMW Men and SMO/SIB Men

	SMW (n = 50)	SMO/SIB (n = 485)
	(percentages)	
None at present	8.0	13.4
Monogamous	6.0	22.5
Several relationship	8.0	6.4
Relationship plus casual[a]	36.0	27.4
Casual sex only	40.0	29.9
NR/DK	2.0	0.4

$\chi^2 = 11.800$ 5 d.f. p = 0.038

Note: a Either one or both partners may be having casual sex.
Source: SAPA Report No. 8.

Characteristics of SMW Men Compared with SMO/SIB Men

In terms of demographic characteristics (structure variables), the SMW sample (n = 50) was not very different from the rest of the sample, 'SMO/SIB' (n = 485). The SMW men differed from the SMO/SIB men in ways that reflect their different lifestyles — they were significantly more likely to have been married, to have had children, to be living with their children (all significant by χ^2 with p < .00005). They also differed in the size of the household they lived in — with a tendency for the SMW men to live in households of three or more and less likely to live in households of size two (p < 0.0002). There were no significant differences between SMW men and SMO/SIB men on any of the other characteristics.

Gay Identity and Lifestyle

One way that SMW men differed from the SMO/SIB men was in their relationship status. Table 10.2 shows the percentages of SMW and SMO/SIB men respectively in different kinds of relationship. Fewer SMW men were in monogamous relationships and more of them were engaging in casual sex, whether they had a relationship as well or not.

Other items relating to sexual identity included information about how their friends saw them and whom they had told about their sexuality. Fewer SMW men than SMO men had told their mother, father, relatives, heterosexual friends, workmates and neighbours about their sexual identity; two of the SMW men (4 per cent) and two of the SIB men (11.8 per cent) said they had told no one. Heterosexuality was attributed more often to the SMW men.

Taken as a whole, these data indicated that there was a tendency for SMW men to be less disclosing of their sexuality. This may be because they were less comfortable with their sexuality, but it could also be because there is less need for them to disclose it — they can 'pass' for being heterosexual very easily. Having been married, or having sexual partners who are women, makes it far more likely that friends, relatives, workmates (even wives) would take their 'normality' for granted. Data also indicated that SMW men did not differ from other men in the sample with respect to the age at which they became aware of their sexual identity. There was, however, a slight tendency for them to be less positive about their sexual identity. It is possible that this made them more reluctant to disclose their sexual identity to relatives and friends. Further information relating to gay identity comes from items regarding involvement with the gay community.

Attachment to Gay Community

In general, the SMW men were much less closely connected with the gay community. Although not statistically significant, SMW men were less likely to say that most or all of their male friends were gay; a much higher percentage of SMW men said that none or only a few of their male friends were gay (or did not respond to the question). They were less likely to belong to gay organizations, to go to meetings, to find their social contacts among gay men. The groups were compared with respect to mean scores on the three measures of attachment to gay community which have been described in Chapter 9. These comparisons are shown in Table 10.3. From these data it can be seen that the SMW men were significantly less attached to the gay community with respect to their social and political activities. They were, however, significantly more likely to seek sexual partners in a wide variety of settings. When the individual items contributing to the sexual engagement scale were examined, it was found that the SMW men were significantly more likely to seek sexual partners at their workplace, at beats and at sex cinemas. It is possible that the higher score of these men on the Sexual Engagement Scale reflects only their wider choice of sex partners, that is, that their sex partners include both men and women. In addition, the SMW men were about twice as likely as SMO/SIB men (12 per cent compared with 5.5 per cent) to have paid for sex with men during the previous twelve months.

Table 10.3. SMW Men Compared with SMO/SIB Men on Three Scales Relating to Gay Community (means, standard deviations and p-values for tests of significance using t-test).

	SMW (n = 50)	SMO/SIB (n = 435)[a]	p
Social Engagement			
Mean:	17.680	19.190	0.000
SD:	3.467	2.306	
Community Attachment			
Mean:	30.880	32.763	0.015
SD:	5.947	5.105	
Sexual Engagement			
Mean:	27.300	24.969	0.001
SD:	4.904	4.405	

Note: a Sample size is reduced because of missing data.
Source: SAPA Report No. 8.

Table 10.4. Number of Casual Partners in the Past Six Months and Frequency of Sex with Casual Partners in the Past Month for SMW and SMO/SIB Men with Multiple Partners

	SMW (n = 42)	SMO/SIB (n = 309)
	(percentages)	
Number of casual (male) partners in the past six months:		
NR/DK	4.5	4.5
None	2.4	0.6
One	4.8	4.2
2–10	45.2	47.9
11–50	35.7	38.5
More than 50	7.1	4.2
	$\chi^2 = 1.12$, 5 d.f. $p = 0.891$	
Frequency of sex with casual partners in the past month:		
NR/DK	7.1	5.2
None	7.1	11.0
1–5 times	50.0	58.3
6–15 times	26.2	21.0
>16 times	9.5	4.6
	$\chi^2 = 5.164$, 4 d.f. $p = 0.457$	

Note: This table refers to those with multiple partners.
Source: SAPA Report No. 8.

In terms of sexual activity, SMW men had about the same number of male casual partners in the past six months as did SMO/SIB men with multiple partners, and had had similar frequency of sex with casual partners in the past month, as shown in Table 10.4.

In general, although their sexual histories in terms of number of casual male partners did not differ from those of the remainder of the sample, these results indicated that SMW men sought sexual partners in a wider variety of contexts than did other gay men. The pattern of results suggests that it is precisely the lack of social and political involvement with the gay community that underlies the wider variety of contexts in which sexual partners are sought.

Sexual Practices

The questionnaire listed a large number of sexual practices and asked for each whether the respondent engaged in it with their male partners, both casual (male) and regular (male) partners. In the comparisons that follow, SMW men were once again compared with the remainder of the sample (SMO/SIB). Table 10.5 shows the percentage of each group that engaged in each practice (either occasionally or frequently). Since some men had regular partners only, some had casual partners only, and some had both regular and casual partners, the number from which some of the percentages are calculated was quite small.

Very few statistically significant differences were found (by χ^2 test) between the two groups. There were significant differences (p = 0.024 and p = 0.048 respectively) between SMW men and SMO men in the percentage who practised 'receptive anal intercourse without a condom' and 'insertive anal intercourse with a condom' with a *regular* partner. In addition, significantly fewer SMW men reported dry kissing with a regular partner (p = .00002). Since the number of SMW men with a regular partner was so small (n = 17), it would be unwise to attach too much importance to these results. The only difference which approached statistical significance with casual partners was in relation to insertive anal intercourse without a condom, where SMW men were slightly more likely to engage in this practice (p = 0.056).

With respect to sex with men, SMW men used condoms about as much as SMO/SIB men did for anal intercourse: 4 per cent never used them, 14 per cent occasionally, 24 per cent often, 28 per cent always and 6 per cent said 'it depends on who'. It may also be compared with the frequency of using condoms in intercourse with women, where 34 per cent never used them, 24 per cent occasionally, 16 per cent often, and 12 per cent used them always. It may also be that some of the men who have never used condoms for intercourse with women have always used them during anal intercourse with men. Such men may have adopted this as a conscious strategy for protecting themselves and their female partners — since they may have judged (probably correctly) that they were more likely to become infected from a man than

Table 10.5. Sexual Practices with Regular and Casual Partners: SMW Men Compared with Remainder (SMO/SIB) of the Sample (p-values for χ^2 tests of significance)

	Regular			Casual		
	SMW (n = 17)	SMO/SIB (n = 292)	p	SMW (n = 42)	SMO/SIB (n = 352)	p
	(percentages)			(percentages)		
Kissing (deep or wet)	88.2	95.0	.228	90.5	83.6	.245
Kissing (dry)	64.7	93.6	.000	90.5	82.2	.174
Rimming (insertive)	41.2	37.0	.730	23.8	20.5	.619
Rimming (receptive)	47.1	39.3	.625	31.0	24.9	.392
Sucking with ejaculation (insertive)	52.9	37.9	.215	40.5	31.8	.258
Sucking with ejaculation (receptive)	35.3	34.1	.916	14.3	19.6	.407
Sucking no ejaculation (insertive)	76.5	85.8	.291	88.1	84.0	.494
Sucking no ejaculation (receptive)	88.2	88.7	.958	83.3	85.5	.707
Fucking without condom (insertive)	35.2	45.9	.393	38.1	24.4	.056
Fucking without condom (receptive)	17.6	45.7	.024	28.6	18.5	.118
Fucking with condom (insertive)	64.7	40.4	.048	61.9	50.1	.149
Fucking with condom (receptive)	47.1	41.8	.669	45.2	42.7	.757
Fucking no ejaculation (insertive)	35.3	39.4	.739	35.7	29.1	.373
Fucking no ejaculation (receptive)	29.4	37.7	.491	31.0	26.3	.519
Mutual masturbation	100.0	93.3	.269	95.2	90.1	.279
Fisting (insertive)	17.6	7.6	.143	9.5	8.8	.882
Fisting (receptive)	11.8	5.4	.279	7.1	4.6	.460
Finger-fucking (insertive)	58.8	53.4	.662	50.0	42.3	.340
Finger-fucking (receptive)	53.7	52.9	.949	50.0	39.8	.206
Sensuous touching	94.1	92.9	.847	97.6	96.0	.609

Source: SAPA Report No. 8.

from a woman. Some were undoubtedly having unprotected anal intercourse with men and unprotected vaginal intercourse with women at least some of the time. No clear pattern of usage of condoms with men and with women emerged from the data. There was great variety in the way men responded to the two questions regarding condoms in intercourse with women and condoms in anal intercourse with men. Condoms were used more often with men than with women.

Three scales relating to sexual practice were developed (see Chapter 5). These were the Essentially Anal Practices (EAP) scale, which

Table 10.6. *Comparisons of SMW Men and SMO/SIB Men on Three Scales of Sexual Practice* (means, standard deviations and p values by t-test)

		SMW (n = 50)	SMO/SIB (n = 485)	p
Anal Practices				
(EAP)	Mean:	3.36	3.71	0.345
	SD:	2.54	2.46	
Oral/Tactile Practices				
(OTP)	Mean:	4.88	5.40	0.014
	SD:	1.97	1.34	
Infrequent Esoteric Practices				
(IEP)	Mean:	0.66	0.77	0.623
	SD:	1.54	1.32	

Source: SAPA Report No. 8.

included the various forms of rimming, anal intercourse (with or without condoms) and finger-fucking; a scale called Oral-Tactile Practices (OTP), which included oral-genital sex, kissing, touching; and the Infrequent Esoteric Practices (IEP) scale, which included infrequent practices such as fisting, bondage and watersports. The mean scores on these scales for SMW men were compared with those of SMO/SIB men using t-tests. Table 10.6 shows the means, standard deviations and p levels for these comparisons.

The groups did not differ significantly on either the EAP or the IEP scale scores. There was, however, a significant difference on the OTP scale scores, with SMW men having a significantly lower (p = 0.014) mean score on this scale. The low incidence of regular partners among the SMW men may account for their lower mean scores. Men in regular relationships had generally higher scores on this scale. This result partially agrees with that of Frazer *et al.* (1988) who found that significantly fewer bisexual men than homosexual men practised kissing, mutual masturbation, oral-genital and oral-anal sex, and insertive anal intercourse. The first three of these practices form part of the OTP scale. Note that the SMW men in the SAPA study did not differ from the remainder of the men with respect to oral/anal sex and insertive anal intercourse.

In terms of education about safe sex practices, and in view of the fact that the SMW men were connected to the gay community through sexual contact rather than social contact, we examined some aspects of their relationships with their casual male partners. SMW men were more likely than SMO/SIB men who have multiple partners to know very little about their male partners. This result approached statistical significance ($\chi^2 = 9.323$, 4 d.f. p = 0.053). This suggests that the contexts in which sex is practised may make it difficult for these men to negotiate safe sex either for their own protection or for their partner's protection.

The number of casual male sex partners in the past six months and the frequency of sex with casual partners in the past month did not differ significantly between SMW men and SMO/SIB men with multiple partners. By definition, SMW men were having sex with both men and women; nevertheless, the kind of sex they practised with men was by and large the same as that practised by men who have sex only with men. Where differences exist, with respect to oral and tactile practices, they can be accounted for by the difference in relationship status already noted — they were more likely to be having casual sex only or to be in a relationship plus casual sex.

Sex with Women

With respect to male sexual partners, the questionnaire asked, regarding each sexual practice, whether the respondent enjoyed it, whether he practised it with casual and with regular partners, and whether he judged it to be safe with respect to transmitting AIDS. In the section of the questionnaire relating to sex with women, respondents were asked only about enjoyment and about safety. Thus we have no information about which practices were actually practised, nor whether the female partners concerned were regular or casual. The data in Table 10.7 came from the 'enjoyment' questions. Data are presented for the fifty SMW men (i.e., men who have had sex with a woman in the past six months). The great majority of the sample did not respond to these items.

The men were asked what two practices were most physically satisfying with women and which were most emotionally satisfying. The most physically satisfying were vaginal intercourse (74 per cent mentioned as one of the two most physically satisfying), oral/genital contact (34 per cent) and sensuous touching (32 per cent). The most emotionally satisfying were vaginal intercourse (68 per cent) and sensuous touching (42 per cent). When asked to rate the importance of vaginal intercourse, 38 per cent rated it as 'very important' and a further 30 per cent as 'quite important'. By comparison, anal intercourse with women was rated as 'very important' by only 12 per cent and 'quite important' by a further 26 per cent.

These data, together with the data about what these men practise

Sustaining Safe Sex

Table 10.7. Enjoyment of Sexual Practices with Female Partners for SMW Men (percentage of SMW men who found each practice very or quite enjoyable: n = 44)

Kissing (wet or deep)	95.4
Kissing (dry)	90.7
Rimming	31.8
Vaginal intercourse (no condom)	88.6
Vaginal intercourse (with condom)	60.4
Vaginal intercourse without ejaculation	45.5
Anal intercourse (no condom)	30.4
Anal intercourse (with condom)	16.3
Anal intercourse without ejaculation	23.3
Oral/genital (fellatio) without ejaculation	75.0
Oral/genital (fellatio) with ejaculation	52.3
Oral-genital (cunnilingus)	65.9
Mutual masturbation	71.7
Sensuous touching	100.0

Source: SAPA Report No. 8.

with male partners, do not support some of the myths about what 'bisexual' men like to do. It has been suggested (Frazer et al., 1988; Bennett, Chapman and Bray, 1989a, 1989b) that such men have sex with men because their female partners were unwilling to satisfy their desire for oral-genital sex. It has also been suggested that it was because the men desire receptive anal intercourse. Neither of these suggestions was supported for this group of men. The SMW men were no more likely than SMO/SIB men to have engaged in receptive anal sex; that is, only a minority engaged in it. They also preferred vaginal to oral sex with women, although they also enjoyed oral-genital sex and found it emotionally and physically satisfying.

A further perception of 'bisexual' men is that they do not tell their female sex partners about their sexual preferences. In this group of SMW men, 58 per cent said that all of their female partners knew that they were 'bisexual' and a further 10 per cent said that some of them did. Only 8 per cent of the SMW men were currently living with a female sexual partner at the time of the study.

In response to a question about why condoms were used for sex with women, 44 per cent stated that they used condoms for contraception, 36 per cent as a protection against AIDS and 36 per cent as a protection against STDs other than AIDS (there is an overlap here: some used them for more than one reason). When asked about acceptability of condoms in sex with women, 26 per cent said they found them 'completely acceptable' and a further 52 per cent 'quite acceptable'. Only 10 per cent said they found them 'unacceptable' (the remainder gave no response to the question).

HIV/AIDS-related Information

Although there was a marginal tendency ($p = 0.051$) for SMW men to have had less contact with the epidemic than the SMO/SIB men, no other differences, including HIV serostatus, approached significance. In general, the SMW men, while not being as closely associated with the gay community in social and political ways, had responded to the epidemic in similar ways to SMO/SIB men in terms of what they knew and the changes they had made. There were no differences when SMW men were compared with the remainder of the sample with respect to mean values on these scales, namely Knowledge of Safe Sex, Knowledge of Unsafe Sex, Pamphlet Awareness, Adoption of Safe Sex, and Relationship Change.

Items in the questionnaire dealing with judged safety of various sexual practices were examined to investigate whether the SMW men judged sex with women to be safer or less safe than sex with men. The sexual practices with men were anal intercourse (insertive and receptive, with and without a condom) and withdrawal (anal intercourse without ejaculation). These were compared with sexual practices with women, namely, vaginal intercourse (with and without a condom) and withdrawal (vaginal intercourse without ejaculation), and anal intercourse (with and without a condom) and withdrawal.

Most of the practices were judged as equally safe or risky with men and women (see Table 10.8). Receptive anal intercourse (not included above because none of the practices with women are analogous to it) was judged as the least safe sexual practice; no one judged receptive anal intercourse without a condom to be more safe than any of the sexual practices involving women. These men were probably correct in believing that receptive anal intercourse for themselves was less safe than any of the (insertive) practices with women.

Conclusion

The group of bisexually active men examined here represents a small but significant minority of men who would otherwise be classified as 'gay' or 'homosexual'. With only one exception, these men had fewer female than male partners — both during their lifetime and during the six months covered by the questions in the survey. Most of them were open with their female sex partners about the fact that they were having sex with men. In addition, we found that many of the remainder

Table 10.8. Percentage of SMW Men Who Judged Practices as More Safe, of Equal Safety or Less Safe with Women Than with Men (n = 44)

	Women more safe	Equal safety	Men more safe
Insertive anal intercourse with men vs vaginal intercourse	25.0	59.1	15.9
Insertive anal intercourse with men vs anal intercourse with women	11.4	59.1	29.5
Insertive anal intercourse with men using a condom vs vaginal intercourse using a condom	25.0	65.9	9.1
Insertive anal intercourse with men using a condom vs anal intercourse with women using a condom	15.9	68.2	15.9
Insertive anal intercourse with men without ejaculation vs vaginal intercourse without ejaculation	34.1	56.8	9.1
Insertive anal intercourse with men without ejaculation vs anal intercourse with women without ejaculation	15.9	63.6	20.4

Source: SAPA Report No. 8.

of the men in the SAPA study, that is, those who were not at the time of the study having sex with women, had had sex with one or more women during their lifetime. Even in a sample of gay and bisexual men, and largely identifying themselves as gay or homosexual, only a minority had been exclusively homosexual during their lifetime.

These findings must be viewed in the context of the study within which the data were collected. The comparisons made in this report have taken this context into account by comparing the SMW men with the remainder of the sample. The majority of the men in the SAPA study were self-identified as gay or homosexual, and the sample was one in which many men were to a greater or lesser extent attached to a gay community. For some purposes, it might be of importance to compare 'bisexual' men with 'heterosexual' (or exclusively heterosexual) men. This has rarely been done. Kinsey's original study is a partial exception, though much of the discussion of 'bisexuality' in Kinsey's report (Kinsey, Pomeroy and Martin, 1948) was under a subheading in the chapter on homosexual practice.

We have noted that the kind of sex with men practised by the 'bisexual' men in this study did not differ from that of other men who have sex with men. They also did not differ in general in terms of demographic characteristics. Knowledge of HIV/AIDS and safe sex and exposure to educational material such as pamphlets did not differ significantly between SMW and SMO/SIB men. Where SMW men differed from the remainder of the sample was in the places where they sought sexual partners, specifically they were more likely to use beats, sex cinemas and male prostitutes, as well as being more likely to find sexual partners in their workplace. In addition, SMW men knew less about their casual male partners than did the other gay men in the SAPA study. All of this information, with the exception of the information regarding the workplace, suggests that in general the context in which SMW men practised sex with men was a less personal one. Such a context may make the practice of safe sex more problematic for these men than for other gay men (Connell *et al.*, 1990).

In Chapter 9 we stressed the importance of *attachment to gay community* in promoting and supporting safe sexual behaviour. In particular, the use of appropriate and effective strategies for the avoidance of HIV infection was found to be related to such an attachment. Although they did not differ from the SMO/SIB men in the extent to which they had adopted safe sex as measured by our AS scale, the SMW men were found to be significantly less attached to the gay community in terms of social engagement and political/cultural involvement, though they were slightly more likely to use a wide selection of places where they sought sexual engagement. A person who is separated from the social and cultural life of the gay community, while maintaining sexual contact with it, would have social and sexual lives which did not overlap, and may lack social support available to other gay men. The above findings indicate that the group of SMW men examined here was likely to contain some such men.

Some theorists (e.g., Paul, 1984) have likened the status of a bisexual man with that of a half-breed, being accepted neither by the gay community nor by the heterosexual community. Zinik (1985: 11) points out that 'bisexuals can find themselves in a "double closet"; they hide their heterosexual activities from their homosexual peers while at the same time hiding their homosexual activities from their heterosexual peers.' Although we have no direct data on these particular men regarding their acceptance or otherwise by either community, their weaker social and political engagement in gay community may be interpretable in these terms. On the other hand, the fact that data about gay identity, such as their own acceptance of their homosexual behaviour, the age at which they became aware of their sexuality, and their satisfaction with it did not distinguish SMW from SMO men does not support the notion put forward by Paul (1984) that social marginalization is the cause of great stress and insecurity.

In view of the importance that many people attach to this group of men with respect to transmitting HIV from the gay to the heterosexual community, these results suggest that we may not be able to rely solely on the gay community to educate these men regarding safe sex practices. It is worrying to note that many of the SMW men in the SAPA study were engaging in dangerous practices with both men and women. Although only a few of them were known to be HIV seropositive, not all of the seropositive men were practising safe sex all of the time. Bisexually active men may need to be reminded about the need to maintain safe sex practices with women as well as with men. As far as sex with women is concerned, these men may not have the same incentive of self-protection as they do when having sex with men, since they may not regard themselves as being at risk of infection from women. They need to be encouraged to adopt a protective attitude towards their female and male partners, and to be reminded that it is possible to contract the virus from vaginal sex. Possibilities for education exist and need to be expanded, but for some of these men national campaigns aimed at the population as a whole may be the only way to get information to them. Specific information about the need to consider the risk associated with insertive anal intercourse (with either men or women) would appear to be needed.

As researchers and educators we must be careful not to fall into the trap of believing that 'bisexual men' form a group. They are certainly not a closed group as far as sexual partners are concerned — and they are often depicted as dangerous specifically because of this. The variety of bisexual behaviour and the contexts in which sex is enacted need to be taken into account in order to ensure that the spread of HIV infection continues to be controlled. We have made some suggestions (Davis, Klemmer and Dowsett, 1991; Dowsett, 1991) about where to start; e.g., workers at beats, possibly including workers who are themselves bisexual men, messages in sex cinemas, continued support and education for male prostitutes, and support for the educational initiatives of the gay community generally. In addition, we suggest that if there is a group of men who are marginalized with respect to both heterosexual and gay communities insofar as their sexual and social worlds do not intersect, it may be necessary to research and implement with great care new strategies for education.

Chapter 11

Five Years On . . .

Before we draw the findings of the SAPA study together, there is one more chapter to write. Although at the time of the SAPA survey we had not planned to reinterview the men, we did so some four to five years later, in 1991. The focus of the follow-up was sexual practice. Our major question was whether the adoption of safe sexual practice and other changes that the SAPA men reported they had made in response to HIV and AIDS had been sustained. The follow-up survey, the Sustaining Safe Sex study (SSS), focused on the question of maintenance and provided information about the stability of the men's sexual responses to HIV/AIDS.

One hundred and forty-five homosexually active men who had taken part in the SAPA survey were reinterviewed. The findings indicated that the majority of men had maintained the changes they had made in 1986/87, some reported further changes to their sexual practice in the direction of 'safe' sex, while a small number reported that they were practising 'unsafe' sex. It appeared that they had 'relapsed'.

'Safety' and 'Relapse'

The issue of maintenance and sustaining safe sex raises questions about definitions of 'safety' and 'relapse'. In 1991 we adopted the following usage: the term 'unsafe' sex refers to sexual practices, abstracted from the context of their enactment, which currently are deemed unsafe in terms of transmission of HIV. Thus, for example, 'unsafe' sex refers to unprotected anal intercourse, while 'safe' sex includes sexual practices such as masturbation and kissing. Debate continues with regard to the safety of oral-genital sexual practice, although many, for example the AIDS Councils in each state in Australia, consider oral-genital sex with no semen exchange to be safe.

The term 'relapse' has been used by some researchers (for example, Adib *et al.*, 1991) to refer to a return to 'unsafe' sex: 'relapse' may mean that there has been an atypical episode in an otherwise 'safe' practice; or it may mean that after a period of 'safe' sexual practice there has been a reversion to constant 'unsafe' practice. Other researchers (for example, Ekstrand and Coates, 1990) distinguish between men who return to unprotected anal intercourse following initial behaviour change and those who continually engage in unprotected anal intercourse. In the latter case there is, in the strict sense of the word, no 'relapse'. Still other researchers (Stall and Ekstrand, 1989; Stall *et al.*, 1990) distinguish men who never practise 'safe' sex from men who have 'occasional high-risk sexual relapses', but seem to ignore those whose return to 'unsafe' sexual practice is more permanent. Much of the usage is confusing. Given that the synonyms for 'relapse' include 'revert', 'backslide', 'degenerate', 'regress', we will use the term 're-lapse' to mean the wholesale reversion to 'unsafe' behaviours and the term 'lapse' to refer to occasional 'unsafe' activity.

There is another problem. Although some researchers, for example, Doll *et al.* (1991), have documented that men discuss their sero-status with their sexual partners, particularly their regular partners, most researchers pay little attention to the details of the interpersonal context of sexual behaviour. Further, most of the authors referred to above as well as others (Gold *et al.*, 1991; Adib *et al.*, 1991) fail to distinguish the practice of unprotected anal intercourse within a mutually exclusive and mutually seronegative relationship from the same behaviour between men who either do not know each other's serostatus or know that their respective serostatus is discordant.

While there is continuing debate about the safety of unprotected anal intercourse between seropositive men, the findings of the follow-up to the SAPA study (the SSS study) demonstrated that many men use their concordant serostatus as a means of preventing the transmission of HIV. A new term is needed, therefore, for unprotected anal intercourse (or any other sexual practice) which is safe in a particular context, even though the same activity is deemed 'unsafe' in the abstract. We suggest 'negotiated safety'.

Variations of Method

In 1991, after some difficulties in securing research funds, we went into the field again. To cut costs, the follow-up survey, Sustaining Safe

Sex or 'SSS', was conducted over the telephone. The questionnaire was shortened considerably and took approximately half an hour to administer. The SSS questionnaire included items from the original SAPA questionnaire which described sexual behaviours as well as items which were predictive of changes in sexual practice. Other questions taken from the original SAPA questionnaire were those which had proved important in the SAPA study: contact with the epidemic; place of residence; attachment to gay community; accuracy of knowledge of HIV transmission and safe sex; and HIV test status of self and sexual partner/s. New items which addressed issues of sexual negotiation were also included, as well as items which measured factors likely to be implicated in the maintenance of change, such as the nature of the men's sexual relationships.

The telephone interviews worked well, and we have no reason to believe that there was any systematic variation in the data collected in this manner compared with the face-to-face interviews of the SAPA survey. The telephone afforded the men a greater degree of privacy, and no one withdrew from the interview once they had begun. We did, however, encounter difficulties locating the men who had taken part in the SAPA study.

SSS Sample

Although we had not planned to reinterview the men, we had asked them, at the time of their first interview in 1986/87, if they would be prepared to give us a contact name, address or telephone number. Ninety-one per cent of the men who had taken part in SAPA volunteered. We attempted to contact these men by telephoning those for whom we had numbers, by writing to those for whom we had addresses and by placing advertisements in local and national gay community papers. The response was not as good as we had anticipated (for details, see Kippax *et al.*, 1993); our final SSS sample comprised 145 men, 30.7 per cent of those who had agreed in 1986/87 to a follow-up. The sample was smaller than we had anticipated. The major reason for the low rate was not refusals but the difficulty we had tracing the men; over 50 per cent had moved in the four to five years between interviews.

Sample Comparisons

Because of the low rate, it is important to examine the differences between the men whom we were able to trace and reinterview and those who either had not volunteered for follow-up or we were unable to trace and were not reinterviewed in 1991.

First, the 473 men who had agreed to follow-up in 1986/87 were very similar to those who declined (n = 62). With the exception of place of residence (men who declined were more likely to live outside the Sydney metropolitan region), they did not differ in terms of age, educational status, occupation, income, religion or country of birth. There were differences, however, with regard to gay community attachment. The men who agreed to further research participation were more likely to belong to gay organizations and more likely to be perceived by their friends as gay. They were also more likely to have been tested for HIV.

When we compared the 145 men whom we reinterviewed in 1991 (the SSS sample) with those we did not interview ('the rest', n = 390), some differences did emerge. The following statistically significant differences are derived from comparisons based on the data collected in 1986/87: at the time of the original survey the men who were reinterviewed in 1991 compared with the men who were not reinterviewed were older (p < 0.0004); they were less likely to be employed in sales or manual jobs (p < 0.0008); they had higher incomes (p < 0.002); they were less likely to test HIV positive (p < 0.04); and they were more likely to be members of gay organizations (p < 0.02). They did not, however, differ from those we did not reinterview with regard to nationality, religious beliefs, educational status, place of residence and self- or others' perception of their sexual identity.

These differences between those men we interviewed in the SSS follow-up and those not interviewed raise questions about the generalizability of the results. The differences indicate that the men who were reinterviewed in 1991 may have been more 'settled' (in the sense of being older and in higher status and better paid occupations) than those who were not. It would be a mistake, therefore, to generalize the results of this follow-up study to young men who have sex with men, or to working-class men.

The difference in HIV status (Table 11.1) is also of concern, and it is difficult to estimate its effect with regard to generalizability. It is possible, however, to rule out some interpretations. Most importantly, the finding that there were fewer men who tested HIV positive among those who were reinterviewed when compared with 'the rest' can *not* be explained in terms of 'unsafe' sexual practice. The SSS sample in 1986/87 were almost indistinguishable from 'the rest' of the original SAPA sample when measured in terms of frequency of 'unsafe' sexual

Table 11.1. *Comparison of HIV Status: 1986/87 and 1991*

	SSS 1991 (n = 145)	Rest 1986/87 (n = 390)
	(percentages)	
No test (n = 174)	29	34
Positive (n = 91)	12	19
Negative (n = 270)	59	47

Source: Kippax *et al.* (1993)

activity.[1] The difference in HIV status may be a function of a reluctance on the part of some of the seropositive men to be reinterviewed, or the death of some of the seropositive men in the four to five years between the original SAPA study and the SSS follow-up.

Because of the sample differences outlined above, the results focus on the 145 men who were reinterviewed (the SSS sample). We compare their responses in 1986/87 with their responses in 1991 in order to assess any changes that they may have made in the intervening years. Where appropriate, we also compare the responses of these 145 men with the total original SAPA sample (n = 535).

At both the initial and 1991 interviews the men provided a detailed description of their sexual behaviour within both regular and casual relationships. They also reported on changes that they had made in order to avoid HIV infection. Thus we had two measures of change: the latter which we refer to as 'reported change', and the former which was based on the differences found in nature of sexual relationship and differences in sexual behaviours between 1986/87 and 1991 data.

Reported Changes

As described in Chapter 7, we distinguished two types of sexual practice change: change in the nature of the men's relationships, Relationship Change (RC); and changes in the sexual behaviours in which the men engaged, Adoption of Safe Sex (AS). These are changes which men reported they had made in response to the threat of HIV transmission. We compare the changes reported by 145 men in both the 1986/87 and the 1991 surveys.

1 The differences are as follows: with reference to regular partners, in 1986/87 the SSS sample was less likely to have had anal intercourse with condoms, either insertive or receptive, than 'the rest'; and with reference to casual partners, the SSS sample was less likely to have engaged in anal intercourse with withdrawal, either insertive or receptive. There was no difference between the samples with respect to anal intercourse without condoms with either regular or casual partners.

Table 11.2. Mean Scale Scores on Relationship Change (RC) and Adoption of Safe Sex
(AS), 1986/87 and 1991

| | Initial sample 1986/87 | | Follow-up sample 1991 | |
	Mean	Standard deviation	Mean	Standard deviation
RC (n = 145)	3.4	2.8	3.5	2.8
AS (n = 145)	24.0	2.1	23.2	2.6

As shown in Table 11.2, the reported change in the nature of the men's relationships as measured by the RC scale was constant over time, as was the change in sexual behaviour as measured by the AS scale. These data confirm the finding above that the majority of men have adopted safe sex and are continuing to practise safe sex.

Factors Affecting Reported Changes

In our analysis of the 1986/87 data reported in Chapter 7, we found that the best predictors of changes, as measured by the Adoption of Safe sex (AS) and Relationship Change (RC), were knowledge of HIV transmission, place of residence and attachment to gay community, and number of years of education. One other variable, degree of contact with the epidemic, was also implicated in the changes documented in this study.

In 1986/87 the adoption of 'safe' sex (AS) was strongest among the 145 men who had comparatively more years of education, stronger sexual and social engagement in gay community, and who were not in monogamous relationships. Although neither locale nor Knowledge of Unsafe Sex (KUS) were significant factors, the overall pattern for the 145 men was similar to that which obtained for the 535 men in 1986/87.

The linear regression analysis on the 1991 data of the same 145 men told a different story. The best predictors of the Adoption of Safe sex (AS) were locale and relationship status (R^2 = 31.6 per cent). The greatest reported change occurred among men in the Extra-metropolitan areas. These men, when compared with men from Inner Sydney, had moved to adopt safe sexual practices. In 1991, as in 1986/87, being in a monogamous relationship, as well as not being in a relationship, was negatively associated with the uptake of safe sexual practice. Engagement in gay community in 1991 was not associated with the uptake of 'safe' sexual practice; nor was Knowledge of Unsafe Sex (KUS).

Table 11.3. Mean Scale Scores on Adoption of Safe Sex Scale by Locale, 1986/87 and 1991

| | Adoption of Safe Sex | | | |
| | 1986/87 | | 1991 | |
Locale in 1986/87	Mean	Standard deviation	Mean	Standard deviation
Inner Sydney (n = 62)	24.32	1.78	23.64	3.07
Northern Suburbs (n = 12)	23.83	1.70	23.33	2.42
Outer-Sydney suburbs				
(n = 12)	24.25	1.48	23.50	2.47
Extra-metropolitan (n = 9)	23.78	1.30	23.78	1.30
ACT (Canberra) (n = 14)	23.79	1.72	22.93	2.09

| | Adoption of Safe Sex | | | |
| | 1986/87 | | 1991 | |
Locale in 1991	Mean	Standard deviation	Mean	Standard deviation
Inner Sydney (n = 68)	24.31	1.77	23.57	3.01
Northern Suburbs (n = 9)	23.89	1.62	23.44	1.81
Outer-Sydney suburbs				
(n = 11)	24.09	1.45	23.27	2.45
Extra-metropolitan (n = 7)	23.86	1.46	24.71	1.89
ACT (Canberra) (n = 15)	23.80	1.66	23.00	2.04

These data are difficult to interpret. The lack of any significant relationship between engagement in gay community, education and knowledge of unsafe sex, on the one hand, and the adoption of safe sex, on the other, may be a function of a ceiling effect. That is, by 1991 the educational message about the adoption of safe sex had spread to nearly all the men in the sample. The one finding that does not fit this interpretation is that the men living in Extra-metropolitan NSW, when compared with men living in Inner Sydney in 1991, had made greater moves in adopting 'safe' sex as measured by the AS scale (see Table 11.3). It is possible that the Inner Sydney men, being those who were among the first to adopt safe sex, are finding it hard to sustain. Or it may be that the Inner Sydney men had found that one practice, the use of condoms, is sufficient and no longer felt the need to adopt other safe sex practices; such a pattern of 'safe' sex would result in a lower score than a pattern where a number of 'safe' sexual practices had been adopted. The data in Table 11.3 indicate that with the exception of the Extra-metropolitan locale, men in all locales, whatever the year, had lower scores on the AS scale in 1991.

We now turn to Relationship Change (RC). The multiple regression analysis of data from the 145 men from the 1986/87 sample indicated that a lack of knowledge of safe sex (KSS), a low level of education, and living in Extra-metropolitan NSW were significantly associated with relationship change, as measured by the RC scale. This result is the same as that reported in Chapter 7 for the entire sample of 535 men.

The regression analysis on the same 145 men, but on the 1991 data, indicated that relationship change was significantly associated with a lack of knowledge of safe sex. There was also a tendency for those with high knowledge of unsafe sex and those with low scores on the Gay Community Attachment scales to turn to relationship change as a means of preventing HIV transmission (R^2 = 29.2 per cent). Although in 1991 there was a higher level of knowledge of safe sex among the men, lack of knowledge of safe sex was related to reported change in relationships, such as moves to monogamy and reduction in the number of casual partners. Locale was not related to relationship change in 1991, although a significant relationship was found in 1986/87. These data point to a more general move on the part of men to change the nature of their relationships in 1991. Again, however, the changes are slight (see Table 11.2) and a ceiling effect is probable.

In general, these data point to the maintenance of changes — in both sexual behaviour and in relationship patterns. What they suggest is that the reported adoption of safe sex, as measured by AS, had been sustained but had not increased — with the exception of men in Extra-metropolitan NSW. Reported relationship change had also not increased but had been sustained and as in 1986/87 was more likely to have been adopted as a prevention strategy by those who have little attachment to gay community and who know least about safe sexual practice, and by those who know most about unsafe sexual practices. As in 1986/87, none of the following variables was significant in predicting change: contact with the epidemic, test status, age.

Changes over Time

We now turn from reported change to differences between the sexual practices of men in 1986/87 and in 1991. Here we compare the data from the 145 men who took part in both surveys.

The men's relationships were classified in the same way as they were in 1986/87. The SSS sample did not differ appreciably from those who were not reinterviewed ('the rest') with regard to the nature of their sexual relations (Table 11.4). Nor was there a significant change between 1986/87 and 1991 when the men were compared as a group

Table 11.4.   *Comparison of Sexual Relationships*

Relationship type	Rest 86/87 (n = 390)	SSS 86/87 (n = 145)	SSS 91 (n = 145)
		(percentages)	
None	13.6	13.1	10.4
Monogamous	20.3	22.8	25.5
Regular plus	27.4	30.3	25.5
Several relationships	7.2	4.8	5.5
Casual only	31.5	29.0	33.1

Source: Kippax *et al.* (1993).

(p > 0.05). Although at the individual level, there was quite considerable movement in and out of relationships (for example, there were
almost as many men moving into monogamy as out of it, and out of
casual-only partnerships as into them), relational patterns remained
reasonably consistent over time. Sexual behaviour within this stable
pattern of relationships did, however, change between 1986/87 and
1991. We report first on the cross-sectional data before turning to the
longitudinal data.

In general, although there were changes to particular sexual behaviours, particularly and importantly with respect to anal intercourse,
there was not a large-scale change in the overall patterning of sexual
practice. Most men engaged in a variety of anal sexual practices and in
a variety of oral and tactile practices in 1986/87 and in 1991.

Between 1986/87 and 1991 there were no net changes in kissing,
sensuous touching and mutual masturbation. Over 90 per cent of
men had engaged in these practices in the six months before 1986/87
and before 1991 with their regular or casual partners. There were also
no changes in fisting, sado-masochistic practices and urolangia
('watersports'); between 5 and 10 per cent of the men had engaged in
these minority practices in the six months prior to being surveyed in
1986/87 and in 1991.

There were small changes, however, with regard to oral-genital
sex, in particular, oral-genital contact with semen exchange. Also there
were changes with regard to oral-anal contact and fingering the rectum.
Between 1986/87 and 1991 there was an increase in the proportion
of men who engaged in these practices. There were also changes with
regard to anal intercourse, and the prevailing trend was in the direction
of safety. There was an increase in the proportion of men who engaged
in anal intercourse with condoms and concomitant decreases in the
proportion of men who engaged in anal intercourse without condoms

and anal intercourse with withdrawal. The decrease was particularly marked in the case of unprotected anal intercourse with casual partners.

Longitudinal Data

These cross-sectional data, while indicating that increasing proportions of men were engaging in safe sexual practices, do not necessarily mean that those who initiated safe sexual practices at one time consistently maintained such behaviours over time. Longitudinal data allow for the clarification of such issues.

The longitudinal data obtained in this study mirror the above cross-sectional findings. Table 11.5 shows the individual changes in sexual practice for men in regular (n = 61 at both times) and casual (n = 73 at both times) relationships in terms of movement away from and towards particular practices. These data indicated that men in *regular* relationships moved away from unprotected anal intercourse, both insertive and receptive. Other practices remained the same with a small but consistent increase in most of the 'safe' practices. The data for sexual practices with *casual* partners showed a similar pattern. As with regular partners, there was significantly less anal intercourse without condoms, but unlike the pattern with regular partners, there was an increase between 1986/87 and 1991 in the number of men who had adopted practices such as fingering the rectum and receptive oral-anal contact, both essentially 'safe' practices.

Most men in the sample had maintained 'safe' or 'unsafe' sexual practice, while others had adopted 'safe' sexual practice between 1986/87 and 1991. A very small number of men had changed their practice in the direction of risk, that is, very few men had 'relapsed'. Overall, the changes that occurred represented a decrease in unprotected or 'unsafe' anal intercourse and an increase in the frequency of some 'safe' oral and tactile practices. The lack of a statistically significant increase in anal intercourse with condoms, either receptive or insertive, with either regular or casual partners, may be explained, at least in part, by the fact that condoms were already being used for anal intercourse in 1986/87 by some of the men (37 per cent with their regular partners and 57 per cent with casual partners).

These data on changes over time indicated that men were, on the whole, adopting 'safe' sexual practices. They also indicated that condom use and the avoidance of unprotected anal intercourse had become the most favoured forms of safe sex — at least among this sample of men. These data strengthen the interpretation offered earlier that the

Table 11.5. Changes in Men's Sexual Behaviours with Regular (Casual) Partners, 1986/87 to 1991

| | Number of men engaging in practice | | | | | |
| | Same | | More | | Less | |
Practice	Reg.	(Cas.)[1]	Reg.	(Cas.)	Reg.	(Cas.)
Wet kissing	42	(37)	7	(16)	10	(20)
Dry kissing	45	(37)	11	(19)	5	(17)
Mutual masturbation	41	(44)	9	(20)	11	(9)
Masturbation in groups	49	(41)	6	(17)	5	(14)
Oral-genital no semen						
(insertive)	34	(35)	12	(21)	15	(16)
(receptive)	39	(35)	6	(21)	16	(17)
Oral-genital with semen						
(insertive)	40	(47)	6	(13)	15	(13)
(receptive)	41	(57)	9	(9)	11	(7)
Fingering the rectum						
(insertive)[2]	30	(34)	16	(29)	14	(9)
(receptive)	29	(38)	17	(23)	14	(11)
Fisting the rectum						
(insertive)	57	(63)	1	(6)	1	(4)
(receptive)	55	(69)	1	(2)	3	(2)
Oral-anal contact						
(insertive)	37	(54)	15	(11)	8	(7)
(receptive)[2]	36	(45)	13	(19)	11	(7)
Anal sex without condoms						
(insertive[2])[2]	37	(53)	3	(5)	21	(15)
(receptive[2])	38	(58)	4	(4)	19	(11)
Anal sex without ejaculation						
(insertive)	43	(53)	6	(6)	12	(14)
(receptive)	36	(58)	9	(5)	16	(10
Anal sex with condoms						
(insertive)	32	(43)	16	(18)	11	(11)
(receptive)	36	(48)	16	(13)	7	(11)
Sensuous touching	50	(46)	5	(14)	6	(13)

Notes: The McNemar test for significance of change with correction for continuity was
used.
1 Refers to type of partner: reg. is regular, cas. is casual.
2 Refers to a statistically significant change, $p < 0.05$, within a regular relationship,
while [2] refers to a statistically significant change, $p < 0.05$, with a casual
partner.
Source: Kippax et al. (1993).

apparent slight reduction in the reported adoption of safe sex practices among Inner Sydney men was a function of these men finding that their adoption of one safe practice, condom use, was sufficient.

Notwithstanding the change towards the adoption of 'safe' sexual practices, the data indicated that some men continued to engage in unprotected anal intercourse, with or without ejaculation — activities which are considered most 'unsafe'. As we shall show below, how-ever, the men who engaged in these activities may not be engaging in 'unsafe' sex — at least in one sense of that term.

Sustaining Safe Sex

Table 11.6. Comparison of 1986/87 and 1991 SSS Sample: HIV Test Status

| | 1991 | | | |
1986/87	Untested	Positive	Negative	Total
Untested	17	2	24	43
Positive	—	15	2[1]	17
Negative	2[2]	5	78	85
Total	19	22	104	145

Note: 1 These two people were either false positives or wrongly coded in the original survey.
2 These two people were either wrongly coded in either survey, or the respondents chose to indicate that they were untested.
Source: Kippax *et al.* (1993).

Self-report of HIV Antibody Test Status

Among the 145 men in the SSS study there was an increase in the number who had been tested for HIV antibodies. In 1986/87 30 per cent of the sample were untested compared with only 13 per cent in 1991. Although there was a small increase in the number of men reporting that they tested HIV seropositive over time, most men tested seronegative (Table 11.6).

When we examined sexual practices in the context of sexual relations and in the context of knowledge of HIV status, we found that concordance in negative (and positive) serostatus was used as an HIV avoidance strategy by the men in the study. In most cases where men had anal intercourse without condoms, their partners were more likely than not to have the same HIV antibody status. This was especially true for men with *regular* partners (n = 82 in 1991).

The details with regard to anal intercourse *without* condoms for these eighty-two men are as follows:

six of the nine (66.7 per cent) *untested* men did not have anal intercourse without condoms with their regular partners, one did so occasionally with his untested partner, and two did so often with their regular partners of unknown HIV status;

twenty-eight of the fifty-eight (48.3 per cent) *HIV seronegative* men did not have anal intercourse without condoms with their regular partners. Of the thirty HIV seronegative men who did have anal intercourse without condoms with their regular partners, twenty-six (86.7 per cent) had HIV seronegative partners. Three of the men did not know their partner's serostatus, and one man occasionally had unprotected anal intercourse with his HIV seropositive partner;

seven of the fifteen (46.7 per cent) *HIV seropositive* men did not have anal intercourse without condoms with their regular partners. Of the eight who did, six (75 per cent) have HIV seropositive partners, while two occasionally had unprotected sex with their HIV seronegative partners.

The pattern for anal sex *with* condoms was reversed: eight of the nine HIV seropositive men (88.9 per cent) who engaged in anal intercourse with condoms did so with regular partners who were HIV seronegative or of unknown test status.

These data indicate that unprotected anal intercourse was most likely to occur with partners of the same serostatus. While the safety of unprotected anal intercourse between two men of HIV positive serostatus is still disputed, unprotected anal intercourse between men who are both HIV seronegative is safe with regard to HIV transmission. The data also indicate that safety was negotiated between men.

Sexual Negotiation

The majority of men in the sample negotiated their sexual activity. Although no comparative data are available because questions on sexual negotiation were not included in the 1986/87 SAPA questionnaire, the following descriptive data demonstrate the ways in which the men incorporated HIV avoidance strategies into their sexual practice.

Seventy-nine per cent of the men had a 'clear agreement' on sexual practice *within* their regular relationship. The nature of that agreement was split between those who agreed to have unrestricted sex (42 per cent) within the relationship and those who agreed to practise 'safe' sex (54 per cent) within the relationship. Twenty-three of the twenty-eight men (82.1 per cent) who had unrestricted sex had concordant serostatus (twenty-one concordant negative pairs, two concordant positive pairs), while twenty of the thirty-six (55.6 per cent) men who practised 'safe' sex had concordant status. Eighty per cent reported never to have broken this agreement.

Seventy-four per cent of the men had a 'clear agreement' on sexual practice *outside* their regular relationship. This agreement fell into three categories: 39 per cent had an agreement that there was no sex outside the relationship; 36 per cent that 'safe' sex was practised all the time, both inside and outside the relationship; and 23 per cent that 'safe' sex was practised with their casual partners only. Eighty-one per cent reported not to have broken this agreement.

These data point to the importance of sexual negotiation in enabling men to put safe sexual strategies (including using concordance of HIV serostatus) into practice. The strategies protect not only the men in the sample but their partners. Men have adopted a range of strategies to avoid infection. Some men have adopted 'safe' sex; that is, practise only *protected* anal intercourse; others have adopted the strategy of 'negotiated safety' which relies on knowledge of their own HIV antibody status and that of their partners.

Conclusions

With regard to changes in sexual practice between 1986/87 and 1991, there has been over all little movement. Taking the reported change and the change over time, the findings indicated that while there is a small increase in the proportion of men in monogamous relationships, there is also a small increase in the proportion of men engaged in casual relationships only. Further, although there has been a slight contraction of the sexual repertoire, the majority of men have attempted to modify their sexual practices in ways which prevent HIV transmission, rather than forsake sex altogether. Many of the men have adopted safe sexual practices such as using condoms and cutting down on unprotected anal intercourse, while some men have also changed the nature of their relationships — by avoiding casual sex, particularly outside their regular relationships, by reducing the number of their casual sexual encounters, and by avoiding particular places and venues. There is no evidence of any large-scale return to unsafe practices, nor is there any sign of a wholesale abandonment of sex. Rather there is evidence of the adoption of a number of overlapping HIV prevention strategies; some men at some stage in their lives favouring the adoption of condoms, others a move to reduce the number of their casual sexual partners, while still others adopt safe sexual practices outside their major or 'regular' relationship. In general, this move to safety is widespread among the men in this somewhat restricted sample.

While care must be taken not to generalize these findings to other samples and populations, in particular, to young or working-class gay and bisexual men, these findings are significant in three important respects.

First, they point to the need to assess the safety or otherwise of sexual practice within the context of sexual partnerships and relationships. Men in this study had changed their sexual practice in the direction of safety. Many adopted condom use, others excluded unprotected anal intercourse from their sexual repertoires, and others took up safe oral and tactile practices. Furthermore, the vast majority of men who were practising so-called 'unsafe' sex did so with partners of the same serostatus. Men of seronegative status who have unprotected anal intercourse with a partner of the same serostatus are, technically speaking, not doing anything unsafe with regard to HIV transmission.

Second, it is important to distinguish the negotiated and agreed practice of unprotected anal intercourse between two partners of HIV negative serostatus from the practice of unprotected anal intercourse between partners where there has been no negotiation and no agreement. The former, which we refer to as 'negotiated safety', should not be interpreted as 'relapse'.

Although it is undoubtedly true that men occasionally break their negotiated agreement, there was little evidence for relapse in the sense of a wholesale reversion to unsafe sex among the men who took part in this study. There were occasional moments of unsafe sex, 'lapses', but such moments do not constitute relapse.

Third, the findings indicate that the educational programs undertaken by the gay community and other organizations have, to a very large extent, been successful. Men in this sample were extremely well informed about which sexual activities are 'safe' and which not. Almost all the gay and bisexual men in this sample had adopted safe sex in some guise or other.

Chapter 12

Personal Strategies,
Collective Responses

As the gay community was an integral part of the whole research process, the findings of our research have credibility and utility in understanding responses to HIV/AIDS, and in framing appropriate education/prevention programs. This is the outcome of our reflexive research strategy.

Personal Prevention Strategies

The response of homosexually active men to the threat of HIV and AIDS was extraordinary. The men we surveyed in New South Wales in 1986/87 and again in 1991, whether they were gay or bisexual or men who self-identified as heterosexual, had changed their sexual practices in order to protect themselves and their sexual partners. We believe that what we were able to document in this period is one of the most profound changes of practice ever found in the social science and public health literature.

One way to capture part of this change and summarize the findings of the SAPA study and the SSS follow-up is to present a picture of the HIV prevention strategies adopted by various groups and individuals in response to HIV and AIDS. The prevention strategies which the men in the studies adopted can be described as follows:

A changes to sexual practice: condom use, avoidance of anal penetrative sex, and the adoption of safe forms of sexual expression;

B changes to nature/type of sexual relationships: reduction in the number of casual partners, reliance on 'regular' partner/s or monogamy;

C negotiated safety: reliance on partner's sexual and drug use history, reliance on concordance of negative HIV antibody status;

D avoidance: avoidance of certain sorts of partners, selection of 'clean' partners.

This classification of four types of strategy does not exhaust the possibilities, but they are the ones most often adopted by the men in their response to HIV and AIDS. Many of the strategies have been advocated in national and targeted educational campaigns, others have been contained in newspaper and other media presentations and reports, and still others have been created by men over time in response to their own experience.

What we documented in the SAPA study and the follow-up SSS study was *part* of a distinctive, diverse and changing response to HIV. In their attempts to make sense of what was happening to them — to their acquaintances, friends, lovers, to their social groups and communities — men modified and transformed their sexual practice. They did this by appropriating the information from the media, particularly the gay press, and modifying the messages as they took account of their own and their friends' understandings of what it means to be gay, in the contexts of their interpersonal and social relationships. The men's personal responses collectively constituted the responses of communities and organizations; and in turn the responses of the organized community reproduced and transformed the personal responses. AIDS Councils were set up, social support systems put in place, education campaigns planned and executed, posters printed, and peer educators and outreach workers funded. The SAPA project itself was part of this organized response. Over the ten years between 1982 and 1992 a culture, and the practices which constituted it, transformed itself.

Knowledge is a necessary condition for change. It is not, however, sufficient; nor does it bring about change in a linear or unitary manner. The findings of our research indicate that community and cultural acceptance, and subsequent changing normative structures within community, as well as the interpersonal social and sexual contexts of men's lives, reshaped and modified the information they received about HIV prevention. The information, too, was not all of a piece and varied depending on its source.

Although in the SAPA and SSS samples the overall level of knowledge about HIV was both accurate and widespread, gay community attached men and men who lived close to centres of gay community had a higher level of accurate information about which practices were safe. These men had greater access to gay community-produced and AIDS organization education campaigns material and information, and they considered AIDS organization and gay community sources important to them.

The negative relationship between accurate knowledge of safe and unsafe sexual practices signalled the non-singularity of response. Men who are secure in their sexual identity and have the support of others like themselves are less cautious in their interpretation of information than men who are separated from gay community or insecure in their sexual identity and practice. A safe sex regime is easier to sustain if others with whom one interacts, both socially and sexually, support that regime.

The 'change in sexual practice' strategies (A), which are generally considered the safest of the prevention strategies, are dependent on accurate knowledge of HIV transmission and ways to prevent it. These A strategies also have to be negotiated in some way — either verbally or non-verbally — within a sexual partnership. Not surprisingly, our data indicated that gay and bisexual men who live within the network of informed social support found it easier to adopt these prevention strategies. There is a consistent trend with regard to condom use: in general, gay community attached men are more likely than non-gay community attached men to use condoms, particularly with casual sexual partners. Men with little gay community attachment are more likely to avoid anal intercourse. The results of the longitudinal study indicated that men, on the whole, have sustained strategies listed under A. They have avoided unprotected anal intercourse, either by avoiding the practice itself or by using condoms. This is not just a reduction of sexual activity generally; there have not been similar reductions in practices which are generally considered safe or 'small risk'.

The 'change in relationships' strategies (B), involving a move to monogamy (or regular partnerships with a reduction in casual partnerships, or no casual sex), have been adopted by some homosexually active men. Both gay community attached men and non-gay community attached men reported moving into monogamous relationships since becoming aware of HIV and AIDS. These strategies (B) are not effective in and of themselves — at the personal level — but they are practised and relied upon by many. Men not attached to gay community and living outside the urban centres of Sydney and Canberra were more likely to rely on these strategies.

Early mainstream press reports focused on monogamy as a guarantee of safety. This is a dangerous strategy for a person to adopt. Its early prominence may derive from epidemiological arguments which correctly state that monogamy is an effective population strategy. Not only is it a dangerous personal strategy because of the possibility of infection within one relationship, but also because of the evidence that relationship patterns among the men in the studies were not stable. Being in a regular relationship was associated with a very high level of unprotected anal intercourse *within* the relationships of the men in the SAPA and SSS studies.

The 'negotiated safety' strategies (C) are very similar, at least superficially, to the 'relationship change' strategies. They, too, carry some risks to the partners, and their effectiveness is dependent on concordant negative serostatus and honesty and trust. The finding that men in regular relationships practised a high level of unprotected anal intercourse, referred to above, may be interpreted another way. When in the SSS study we investigated further, we found that many men in regular relationships practise what we have called 'negotiated safe sex'; they have unprotected anal intercourse with their regular partner of the same HIV antibody status and reach a variety of agreements about sex outside the relationship (typically 'no anal intercourse' or 'condoms always'). While the safety of unprotected anal intercourse between two men of HIV positive serostatus is still disputed, unprotected anal intercourse between men who are both HIV seronegative is safe with regard to HIV transmission — given honesty and trust between the sexual partners. That honesty and trust is more likely in long-standing relationships and least likely in casual encounters. Testing for HIV antibody status is, of course, also implicated in this strategy.

Sexual negotiation has an important part to play, particularly within regular relationships. It enables men to put safe sexual strategies (including using concordance of HIV serostatus) into practice. It has been adopted by both gay community attached and unattached men, but it was more likely to be adopted as a strategy by gay community attached men. The latter were more likely than non-gay community attached men to be in regular, although not monogamous, relationships. The distinction between 'monogamous' and 'regular relationships' is an important one: the word 'monogamy' carries with it notions of exclusiveness and fidelity which in some ways preclude negotiation; 'regular', on the other hand, connotes the openness of sexual relationships which in turn allow for negotiation. Also important in this context is our finding that reciprocity typified men's sexual practice.

Both gay community attached and non-gay community attached men reported adopting avoidance strategies (D). These are ineffective strategies and were adopted more often by non-gay community attached men. Their adoption appears to be a function of alienation and anxiety rather than a sensible or well informed response to HIV. Changes like these appear to be associated with vulnerability and are likely to be ill-judged or irrational. These strategies also assume that one is not infected oneself — and that the whole name of the game is avoidance rather than the prevention of transmission. Avoidance strategies, too, feed into discrimination which in turn may reduce the social support among gay men. Both these D strategies and those included under B provide very little protection from the virus.

Two major areas of importance to the social aspects of the prevention of HIV, gay community and the nature of relationships, emerged from our results. A 'safe sex' culture has developed: it is now largely taken for granted that condoms will be used for anal intercourse; it is intercourse *without* condoms that needs to be negotiated, not intercourse *with* condoms. The context, both interpersonal and social, of sexual activity is central to an understanding of sexual practice and its change. It is in these contexts that the meanings that constitute safe sex are negotiated, debated and appropriated.

Collective Responses

Given that patterns of sexual behaviour change indicated that measures of knowledge of HIV transmission and responses to other HIV/AIDS issues were related to social and geographic proximity to an established and observable gay community, in addition to a significant degree of participation in it, it would appear that the reach of the gay community prevention programs has a definite limit. Subsequent research among homosexual working-class men has indicated difficulties concerned with gay community participation and with educational materials produced by gay community programs (Connell *et al.*, 1991; Dowsett, Davis and Connell, 1992a). Educational strategies for reaching men beyond gay community are an obvious need, as are educational strategies which work through existing patterns of interpersonal networks and relationships, and foster group support for change.

Support for such educational strategies comes also from studies other than our own. In May 1989 the World Health Organisation hosted a workshop in Geneva on 'Health Promotion Activities Directed towards Gay and Bisexual Men'. Seven large cities with significant patterns of homosexual HIV transmission — London, New York, San Francisco, Sydney, Paris, Amsterdam and Rio de Janeiro — were represented by researchers, AIDS educators and activists. One task of the researchers was to analyze the impact of the education efforts aimed at gay and bisexual men, and assess what is successful and what could be utilized with other at-risk populations (Mantell, 1989; Aggleton, Coxon and Weatherburn, 1989; Pollak, 1989; Tielman, 1989; Dowsett, 1989a). It was clear that the activities of the gay communities from the various cities had much in common and they had been very successful in reducing the size and impact of the epidemic among their constituents.

That the strategies are working in Australia is confirmed by the following figures. Using the number of AIDS cases per 1,000,000, Australia has fallen from third position in 1986 to sixth position in 1991 when compared with some reasonably similar Western European countries. As in Denmark and the Netherlands (two countries which Australia most resembles with regard to the pattern of HIV transmission), rates of homosexual transmission of HIV, which account for most cases of HIV, appear to be dropping, while there is a small increase in heterosexual transmission. The overall picture is one of a small but steady drop in the HIV infection rate.

What has produced this very welcome fall, and what can we say about education and prevention? Although it is very difficult to pinpoint which prevention program or education campaign, the findings reported here indicate that the government strategy of engaging and funding community groups, including gay community groups, in research and in developing educational policies and programs has been successful. The funding of educational programs in schools and the innovative work of institutions such as the AIDS Councils, and the development of peer-based educational programs, has worked.

In a recent paper (Duckett and van Reyk, 1992) Australia's response to HIV and AIDS has been likened to that of Norway, Denmark and the Netherlands. In all four countries emphasis has been placed on information and education, on consensus and non-coercion, on creating a supportive environment and strengthening community action. In all five countries there have been decreases in HIV infections.

As noted in Chapter 1, we need to move beyond the individualistic emphasis of much official health education and academic AIDS research towards collective, social strategies for change. The aim of such work is not so much to change individual 'attitudes' or 'health behaviours' as to move whole networks and groups of people towards safer practice and encourage the social processes among them which can sustain prevention. The SAPA study, being designed, carried out and disseminated with and for the relevant community, has provided important theoretical insights and empirical evidence regarding these social processes. Although we have documented these processes for one community, the processes themselves are quite general. HIV infection is preventable. The possibility of stopping the epidemic lies in the combination of well crafted public health education programs and grassroots social action.

Changes in Climate

We must not, however, be complacent. The epidemic is not static, nor are responses, personal or collective, to it. A number of things have changed since we began our work in 1986. We shall refer here to those we believe are the most important.

One finding in 1986/87 was that degree of contact with the epidemic was only marginally associated with the adoption of safe sexual practices. Since then, however, there has been a dramatic increase in contact with the epidemic. Most gay and bisexual men in New South Wales now know someone who is infected by HIV. There had also been an increase in the percentage of men who know someone who has died of AIDS, from 67 per cent in 1986/87 to 90 per cent in 1991; and an increase in the percentage of men caring for someone with AIDS, from 24 per cent in 1986/87 to 55 per cent in 1991. Such contact with the epidemic was, in 1991, widespread and certainly not confined to inner Sydney.

It has become increasingly apparent that gay communities themselves are changing as many of the men engaged in these communities become ill. Although the rate of increase of HIV among gay men is declining, the number of men becoming ill with AIDS has markedly increased. There are greater demands on men to care for others, and greater psychological demands on men as their lovers, friends and acquaintances die. There is also a tension developing between those with HIV and those who are not infected. The impact of this change is impossible to gauge; one suggestion is that men will 'give up' and throw safe sex to the winds, another is that it will increase men's efforts to adopt safe sexual practice. Perhaps both will occur as well as responses that we have not yet thought of.

Another change concerns HIV testing. Testing is becoming more and more part of a prevention strategy, although for some time in the early 1980s the AIDS Council and gay community resisted the calls for homosexually active men to be tested. Many gay and bisexual men were tested in that period, and the number has increased. Thirty per cent of the sample were untested in 1986/87 compared with 13 per cent in 1991. Although in 1986/87 testing had a minimal impact on sexual behaviour, knowing one's HIV serostatus appears to be becoming an important part of some men's HIV prevention strategy.

The passing of time produces change. It is now ten years since the diagnosis of the first Australian case of AIDS. People, particularly those men attached to gay community, have become better informed about transmission of HIV, and, at the same time, HIV and AIDS have become part of their world. Men now 25 years old were only 15 years of age when AIDS came to Australia. For such men, HIV has been a part of their experience for most, if not all, of their sexual life. The impact on the young is also difficult, if not impossible, to estimate.

As sexual practices are modified in response to HIV, and as social and cultural practices of gay community respond to the increasing pressure of illness, gay identity and sexuality will be transformed. Talk about AIDS and HIV in schools, the debate about bisexuality and 'men who have sex with men', and the safe sex reminders in the press and on television will feed into this process. Distinctions between gay and bisexual, heterosexual and gay, will become blurred or, perhaps, sharper. Certainly our own understandings and definitions of homosexual, heterosexual, bisexual have changed in the course of doing this research.

A final change concerns the research process itself. As we have noted in Chapter 3, an important part of the research process has been the feedback of the findings to those affected by the epidemic. Men attached to gay community and members of AIDS organizations are acquainted with the results of our enquiry. The research, in turn, has to take account of the dynamics of change. Much of the study in which we are now engaged is focused on the above issues.

Future Directions

Although SAPA Study A is perhaps the best known part of our work in the HIV/AIDS field, it is far from being the whole story. Since SAPA A began, other research programs have developed around it. Three qualitative studies have been carried out using the life-history approach. Community attachment, social class and distance from the organized gay community have been examined in relation to such issues as sexual identity, sexual practices, intimacy and barriers to the adoption of safe sex. Three different samples were used: the inner-Sydney gay community; working-class gay men; and two urban sites outside Sydney. Two other follow-up cross-sectional surveys on men who have sex with men have also been carried out: one on a small sample of men in Tasmania and the other a national survey of over 2500 men. Both surveys used questionnaires based on the original SAPA questionnaire. Two complementary studies are also underway to document the impact of HIV and AIDS on those living with HIV and AIDS, and on gay community. Moments of change in the lives of gay men is another project in which we are involved.

We have also been involved in survey and qualitative research, some of it using a new technique, 'memory-work', with heterosexual men and women. The focus of these studies has been the prevention strategies adopted by men and women, issues concerning the negotiation of safe sex and barriers to the adoption of safe sex strategies. HIV-related discrimination and anti-gay violence have also been the subject of some of our work, and we have been involved in a series of policy and evaluation projects on HIV/AIDS education.

Although the research has overwhelmed our other academic interests and activities, and burnout is a genuine issue, it has been an exciting and rewarding number of years. We have learnt a great deal about the nature of social research and the difficulties of pursuing it in the public health area. The research has strengthened our resolve to pursue more boldly what is distinctively social in the issues surrounding HIV and AIDS. Health education has a great deal to learn and gain from the lessons of HIV and AIDS, in particular with regard to the social aspects of prevention.

It is important to conceptualize change as a collective response. The significance of such a conceptualization lies in its inherent political and educational implications. Attention is focused on the community, on the group, not on the individual or aggregates of individuals, infected or not, high risk or not. People do things in ways which they and others find intelligible, which make sense, a *common sense*. In the non-traditional public health models there is a focus on the promotion of health through the restructuring of social norms in ways which are relevant to the members of communities and groups.

Bibliography

ADIB, S.M., JOSEPH, J.G., OSTROW, D.G. and SHERMAN, A.J. (1991) 'Predictors of Relapse in Sexual Practices among Homosexual Men', *AIDS Education and Prevention*, 3, 4, 293–304.

ADIB, S.M., JOSEPH, J.G., OSTROW, D.G., TAL, M. and SCHWARTZ, A. (1991) 'Relapse in Sexual Behaviour among Homosexual Men: A Two-year Follow-up from the Chicago MACS/CCS', *AIDS*, 5, 757–60.

ADORNO, T.W., FRENKEL-BRUNSWICK, E., LEVINSON, D.J. and SAND-FORD, R.N. (1950) *The Authoritarian Personality*, New York, Harper and Row.

AGGLETON, P.J., COXON, A. and WEATHERBURN, P. (1989) 'AIDS Health Promotion Activities Targeted at Homosexually Active Men in London (UK): A Briefing Document Prepared for the WHO Global Programme on AIDS', Paper to the World Health Organisation Workshop on Health Promotion Activities Directed towards Gay and Bisexual Men, Geneva, 29–31 May.

AIDS COUNCIL OF NEW SOUTH WALES (1992) *Annual Report for 1991–92*, Sydney, AIDS Council of New South Wales.

AJZEN, I. and FISHBEIN, M. (1980) *Understanding Attitudes and Predicting Social Behaviour*, Englewood Cliffs, N.J., Prentice-Hall.

AJZEN, I. and MADDEN, T.J. (1986) 'Prediction of Goal-directed Behaviour: Attitudes, Intentions and Perceived Behavioural Control', *Journal of Experimental Social Psychology*, 22, 453–474.

ALTMAN, D. (1979) *Coming Out in the Seventies*, Sydney, Wild and Woolley.

ALTMAN, D. (1982) *The Homosexualization of America; The Americanization of the Homosexual*, New York, St Martin's Press.

ANDERSON, R.M. and MAY, R.M. (1992) 'Understanding the AIDS Pandemic', *Scientific American*, 266, 5, 20–27.

ANNS, M. (1987) 'HIV Transmission: Factors Affecting Adoption of Low Risk Behaviours', Paper presented at NACAIDS Seminar, Sydney.

AUSTRALIAN BUREAU OF STATISTICS PUBLICATIONS: 'Social Indicators Australia No. 4 1984' (Cat. No. 4101.0); 'Estimated Labour Force (Civilian Population) November 1986' (Cat. No. 6201.1); 'Distribution and Composition of Employee Earnings and Hours — Australia, May, 1986' (Cat. No. 6306.0); 1986 Census, NSW (STE1) and ACT (STE8); Seven-page summaries (format CSCO7): Tables CO1, CO2, C03, C05, C21, C23, C26; Twenty-one page summaries (format CD21) table C64: Microfiche tables CX0014, Cat. No. C86.501.

AUSTRALIAN GONOCOCCAL SURVEILLANCE PROGRAM (1988) 'Changing Patterns in Gonococcal Infections in Australia, 1981–1987', *Medical Journal of Australia*, 149, 609–612.

BALLARD, J. (1989) 'The Politics of AIDS', in GARDNER, H. (Ed.), *The Politics of Health: The Australian Experience*, Melbourne, Churchill Livingstone.

BANDURA, A. (1989) 'Self-efficacy Mechanism in Physiological Activation and Health-promoting Behavior', in MADDEN, J., MATTHYSSE, S. and BARCHAS, J. (Eds), *Adaptation, Learning and Affect*, New York, Raven.

BAUMAN, L.J. and SIEGEL, K. (1987) 'Misperception among Gay Men of the Risk for AIDS Associated with Their Sexual Behavior', *Journal of Applied Social Psychology*, 17, 3, 329–350.

BECKER, M. (Ed.) (1974) *The Health Belief Model and Personal Health Behavior*, Thorofare, N.J., Charles B. Slack.

BECKER, M. and JOSEPH, J. (1988) 'AIDS and Behavioral Change to Reduce Risk', *American Journal of Public Health*, 78, 394–410.

BENNETT, G. and PETHERBRIDGE, A. (1986) *Report on a Survey of Gay Sauna Patrons from the Gay Counselling Service of NSW to ACON*, Sydney, Gay Counselling Service.

BENNETT, G., CHAPMAN, S. and BRAY, F. (1989a) 'Sexual Practices and "Beats": AIDS-related Sexual Practices in a Sample of Homosexual and Bisexual Men in the Western Area of Sydney', *Medical Journal of Australia*, 151, 309–314.

BENNETT, G., CHAPMAN, S. and BRAY, F. (1989b) 'A Potential Source of Transmission of the Human Immuno-deficiency Virus into the Heterosexual Population: Bisexual Men Who Frequent "Beats"', *Medical Journal of Australia*, 151, 314–318.

BOULTON, M. and COXON, T. (1991) 'Bisexuality in the United Kingdom', in TIELMAN, R.A.P., CARBALLO, M. and HENDRIKS, A.C.

(Eds), *Bisexuality and HIV/AIDS*, Buffalo, N.Y., Prometheus Books.

BRANDT, A.M. (1988) 'AIDS and Metaphor: Towards the Social Meaning of Epidemic Disease', *Social Research*, 55, 3, 413–432.

BURCHAM, J.L., TINDALL, B., MARMOR, M., COOPER, D.A., BERRY, G. and PENNY, R. (1989) 'Incidence and Risk Factors for Human Immunodeficiency Virus Seroconversion in a Cohort of Sydney Homosexual Men', *Medical Journal of Australia*, 150, 634–9.

CALDER, B.J. and ROSS, M. (1973) *Attitudes and Behaviour*, New Jersey, General Learning Press.

CALLEN, M. (1983) *How to Have Sex in an Epidemic*, New York, News From the Front Publications.

CAMPBELL, I.M., BURGESS, P.M., GOLLER, I.E. and LUCAS, L. (1986) *A Prospective Study of Psychological Factors Influencing HIV Infection in Homosexual/Bisexual Men*, Unpublished questionnaire, Melbourne, University of Melbourne, Department of Psychology.

CAMPBELL, I.M., BURGESS, P.M., GOLLER, I.E. and LUCAS, L. (1988) *A Prospective Study of Factors Influencing HIV Infection in Homosexual and Bisexual Men. A Report of Findings: Stage I*, Melbourne, University of Melbourne, Department of Psychology.

CAPLAN, P. (1987) *The Cultural Construction of Sexuality*, London, Tavistock.

CARR, A. (1987) 'Report on the Third International AIDS Conference, Washington, June 1987', Melbourne, Victorian AIDS Council.

CARR, A. (1988) *Behaviour Change in Australia in Response to the Threat of HIV Infection 1983–1988: A Survey of Current Knowledge*, Canberra, Commonwealth Department of Community Services and Health.

CARR, A. (1989) 'Gay Men's Relationships and Unsafe Sex', *National AIDS Bulletin*, 3, 5, 27–31.

CHIN, J. (1991) Keynote address presented at the Sixth International Conference on HIV/AIDS, Florence, June.

COATES, T.J., TEMOSHOK, L. and MANDEL, J. (1984) 'Psychosocial Research Is Essential to Understanding and Treating AIDS', *American Psychologist*, 39, 11, 1309–1314.

COMMONWEALTH OF AUSTRALIA (1989) *National HIV/AIDS Strategy. A Policy Information Paper*, Canberra, Australian Government Publishing Service.

CONNELL, R.W. (1987) *Gender and Power*, Cambridge, Polity Press.

CONNELL, R.W. and DOWSETT, G.W. (1992) (Eds) *Rethinking Sex: Social Theory and Sexuality Research*, Melbourne, Melbourne University Press.

CONNELL, R.W. and KIPPAX, S. (1990) 'Sexuality in the AIDS Crisis: Patterns of Sexual Practice and Pleasure in a Sample of Australian Gay and Bisexual Men', *Journal of Sex Research*, 27, 2, 157–98.

CONNELL, R.W., CRAWFORD, J., DOWSETT, G.W., KIPPAX, S., SINNOTT, V., RODDEN, P., BERG, R., BAXTER, D. and WATSON, L. (1990) 'Danger and Context: Unsafe Anal Sexual Practice among Homosexual and Bisexual Men', *Australian and New Zealand Journal of Sociology*, 26, 2, 187–208.

CONNELL, R.W., CRAWFORD, J., KIPPAX, S., DOWSETT, G.W., BAXTER, D., WATSON, L. and BERG, R. (1989) 'Facing the Epidemic: Changes in the Sexual Lives of Gay and Bisexual Men in Australia and Their Implications for AIDS Prevention Strategies', *Social Problems*, 36, 4, 384–402.

CONNELL, R.W., CRAWFORD, J., KIPPAX, S., DOWSETT, G.W., BOND, G., BAXTER, D., BERG, R. and WATSON, L. (1988) *Social Aspects of the Prevention of AIDS: Study A, Report No. 1. Method and Sample*, Sydney, Macquarie University, School of Behavioural Sciences.

CONNELL, R.W., DOWSETT, G.W., RODDEN, P., DAVIS, M., WATSON, L. and BAXTER, D. (1991) 'Social Class, Gay Men, and AIDS Prevention', *Australian Journal of Public Health*, 15, 3, 178–189.

CRAWFORD, J., DOWSETT, G.W., KIPPAX, S., CONNELL, R.W., BAXTER, D., BERG, R. and WATSON, L. (1992) *Social Aspects of the Prevention of AIDS: Study A, Report No. 8. Gay and Bisexual: Bisexual and Gay — The Sexual Behaviour of Men Who Have Sex with Men and Women in an Australian Sample of Gay and Bisexual Men*, Sydney, Macquarie University, School of Behavioural Sciences.

CRAWFORD, J., KIPPAX, S. and DOWSETT, G.W. (1990) 'The Role of Contact with the HIV/AIDS Epidemic in Determining Behaviour Change in a Sample of Homosexual and Bisexual Men', in SOLOMON, P.J., FAZEKAS DE ST GROTH, C. and WILSON, S.R. (Eds), *Projections of Acquired Immune Deficiency Syndrome in Australia Using Data to the End of September 1989*, National Centre for Epidemiology and Population Health, Working Papers, 16, 89–91.

CRIMP, D. (Ed.) (1988) *AIDS: Cultural Analysis, Cultural Activism*, Cambridge, Mass., MIT Press.

DARROW, W.W., JAFFE, H.W., THOMAS, P.A., HAVERKOS, H.W., ROGERS, M.F., GUINAN, M.E., AUERBACH, D.M., SPIRA, T.J. and CURRAN, J.W. (1986) 'Sex of Interviewer, Place of Interview and Responses of Homosexual Men to Sensitive Questions', *Archives of Sexual Behavior*, 15, 1, pp. 79–89.

DAVIES, P.M., HUNT, A.J., MARCOURT, M.P.A. and WEATHERBURN, P. (1990) *Longitudinal Study of the Sexual Behaviour of Homosexual Males under the Impact of AIDS: A Final Report to the Department of Health*, London, Project SIGMA.

DAVIS, M. (1990) 'Peer Education and a Framework for Change in Queensland', *National AIDS Bulletin*, 5, 37–40.

DAVIS, M.D., KLEMMER, U. and DOWSETT, G.W. (1991) *Bisexually Active Men and Beats: Theoretical and Educational Implications* [The Report of the Bisexually Active Men's Outreach Project], Sydney, AIDS Council of New South Wales and Macquarie University, AIDS Research Unit, National Centre for HIV Social Research.

D'EMILIO, J. (1983) *Sexual Politics, Sexual Communities*, Chicago, Ill., University of Chicago Press.

DEUTSCHER, M. (1983) *Subjecting and Objecting*, St Lucia, Qld, University of Queensland Press.

DICLEMENTE, R.J., BOYER, C.B. and MILLS, S.J. (1987) 'Prevention of AIDS among Adolescents: Strategies for the Development of Comprehensive Risk-reduction Health Education Programs', *Health Education Research*, 2, 3, 287–291.

DICLEMENTE, R.J., ZORN, J. and TEMOSHOK, L. (1987) 'The Association of Gender, Ethnicity and Length of Residence in the Bay Area to Adolescents' Knowledge and Attitudes about Acquired Immune Deficiency Syndrome', *Journal of Applied Psychology*, 17, 3, 216–230.

DOLL, L.S., BYERS, R.H., BOLAN, G., DOUGLAS, J.M., MOSS, P.M., WELLER, P.D., JOY, D., BARTHOLOW, B.N. and HARRISON, J.S. (1991) 'Homosexual Men Who Engage in High-risk Sexual Behaviour: A Multicenter Comparison', *Sexually Transmitted Disease*, 18, 170–175.

DONOVAN, B. (1988) 'Social and Behavioural Components of Clinical Studies, in Commonwealth of Australia', in *Living with AIDS: Toward the Year 2000* [Report of the Third National Conference on AIDS, Hobart, 4–6 August], Canberra, Australian Government Publishing Service, pp. 166–71.

DOWSETT, G.W. (1989a) ' "You'll Never Forget the Feeling of Safe Sex!" AIDS Prevention Strategies for Gay and Bisexual Men in Sydney, Australia', Paper to the World Health Organisation Workshop on AIDS Health Promotion Activities Directed towards Gay and Bisexual Men, Geneva, 29–31 May.

DOWSETT, G.W. (1989b) 'Reaching Men Who Have Sex with Men in Australia', Paper presented at the Second International Symposium on AIDS Information and Education, Yaoundé, Cameroon, 22–26 October.

DOWSETT, G.W. (1990) 'Reaching Men Who Have Sex with Men in Australia. An Overview of AIDS Education: Community Intervention and Community Attachment Strategies', *Australian Journal of Social Issues*, 25, 3, 186–198.

DOWSETT, G.W. (1991) *Men Who Have Sex with Men: Considerations for a National HIV/AIDS Educational Intervention*, Briefing paper to the AIDS Policy and Programs Branch, Department of Health Housing and Community Services, Canberra.

DOWSETT, G.W. and DAVIS, M.D. (1992) *Transgression and Intervention: Homosexually Active Men and Beats. A Review of an Australian HIV/ AIDS Outreach Prevention Strategy*, Sydney, Macquarie University, AIDS Research Unit, National Centre for HIV Social Research.

DOWSETT, G.W., DAVIS, M.D. and CONNELL, R.W. (1992a) 'Working-class Homosexuality and AIDS Prevention: Some Recent Research from Sydney, Australia', *Psychology and Health*, 6, 313–324.

DOWSETT, G.W., DAVIS, M.D. and CONNELL, R.W. (1992b) 'Gay Men, HIV/AIDS and Social Research: An Antipodean Perspective', in Aggleton, P., DAVIES, P. and HART, G. (Eds), *AIDS: Rights, Risk and Reason*, London, Falmer Press.

DUCKETT, M. and VAN REYK, P. (1992) 'AIDS: Have We Got It Right? — A View from the Trenches', *National AIDS Bulletin*, 6, 10, 44–47.

EKSTRAND, M.L. and COATES, T.J. (1990) 'Maintenance of Safer Sexual Behaviours and Predictors of Risky Sex: The San Francisco Men's Health Study', *American Journal of Public Health*, 80, 973–977.

ELLIS, H. (1923) *Studies in the Psychology of Sex, Volume 2: Sexual Inversion*, Philadelphia, Pa., Davis (original work published 1897).

EMMONS, C.A., JOSEPH, J.G., KESSLER, R.C., WORTMAN, C.B., MONTGOMERY, S. and OSTROW, D. (1986) 'Psychosocial Predictors of Reported Behaviour Change in Homosexual Men at Risk for AIDS', *Health Education Quarterly*, 13, 4, 331–345.

EPSTEIN, C.F. (1988) *Deceptive Distinctions*, New Haven, Conn., Yale University Press.

ERIKSON, E.H. (1965) *Childhood and Society*, 2nd ed., Harmondsworth, Penguin.

FEE, E. and FOX, D.M. (Eds) (1988) *AIDS: The Burdens of History*, Berkeley, Calif., University of California Press.

FELDMAN, D.A. (1985) 'AIDS and Social Change', *Human Organization*, 44, 343–347.

FISHBEIN, M. and AJZEN, I. (1975) *Belief, Attitude, Intention and Behavior: An Introduction to Theory and Research*, Reading, Mass., Addison-Wesley.

FISHBEIN, M. and MIDDLESTADT, S.E. (1989) 'Using the Theory of Reasoned Action as a Framework for Understanding and Changing AIDS-related Behaviors', in MAYS, V.M., ALBEE, G.W. and SCHNEIDER, S.F. (Eds), *Primary Prevention of AIDS: Psychological Approaches*, New York, Sage Publications.

FISHER, J.D. (1988) 'Possible Effects of Reference Group-based Social Influence on AIDS-risk Behaviour and AIDS Prevention', *American Psychologist*, 43, 11, 914–920.

FITZPATRICK, R., BOULTON, M. and HART, G. (1989) 'Gay Men's Sexual Behaviour in Response to AIDS: Insights and Problems', in AGGLETON, P., HART, G. and DAVIES, P. (Eds), *AIDS: Social Representations, Social Practices*, Lewes, Falmer Press.

FOUCAULT, M. (1980) *The History of Sexuality*, Vol. 1, New York, Vintage.

FRAZER, I.H., MCCAMISH, M., HAY, I. and NORTH, P. (1988) 'Influence of Human Immunodeficiency Virus Antibody Testing on Sexual Behaviour in a "High-risk" Population from a "Low-risk" City', *Medical Journal of Australia*, 149, 365–368.

FREUD, S. (1964a) 'Fragment of an Analysis of a Case of Hysteria', in STRACHEY, J. (Ed. and Trans), *The Standard Edition of the Complete Psychological Works*, Vol. 7, London, Hogarth Press, pp. 1–122, (original work published 1905).

FREUD, S. (1964b) 'Three Essays on the Theory of Sexuality', in STRACHEY, J. (Ed. and Trans), *The Standard Edition of the Complete Psychological Works*, Vol. 7, London, Hogarth Press, pp. 123–243, (original work published 1905).

GAGNON, J.H. (1988) 'Sex Research and Sexual Conduct in the Era of AIDS', *Journal of Acquired Immune Deficiency Disease*, 1, 593–601.

GAGNON, J.H. and SIMON, W. (1974) *Sexual Conduct*, London, Hutchinson.

GIDDENS, A. (1984) *The Constitution of Society*, Cambridge, Polity Press.

GOCHROS, J.S. (1991) 'Bisexuality and Female Partners', in TIELMAN, R.A.P., CARBALLO, M. and HENDRIKS, A.C. (Eds), *Bisexuality and HIV/AIDS*, Buffalo, N.Y., Prometheus Books.

GOEDERT, J.J. (1987) 'What Is Safe Sex? Suggested Standards Linked to Testing for Human Immunodeficiency Virus', *New England Journal of Medicine*, 316, 1339–1342.

GOLD, R., SKINNER, M., GRANT, P. and PLUMMER, D. (1989) 'Situational Factors Associated with, and Rationalizations Employed to Justify Unprotected Intercourse in Gay Men', Paper presented at the Fifth International Conference on AIDS, Montreal, 4–9 June.

GOLD, R.S., SKINNER, M.J., GRANT, P.J. and PLUMMER, D.C. (1991) 'Situational Factors and Thought Processes Associated with Unprotected Intercourse in Gay Men', *Psychology and Health*, 5, 259–278.

GORDON, P. (1989) *Safer Sex Education Workshops and Bisexual Men: A Review*, Unpublished Manuscript prepared for the Health Education Authority, London.

GRAHAM, L. and CATES, J.A. (1987) 'AIDS: Developing a Primary Health Care Task Force', *Journal of Psychosocial Nursing and Mental Health Services*, 25, 12, 21–25.

HABERMAS, J. (1984) *The Theory of Communicative Action*, Vol. 1, Boston, Mass., Beacon Press.

HARRE, R. (1983) *Personal Being*, Oxford, Basil Blackwell.

HART, J. (1985) 'Social Aspects of AIDS', *Australian Journal of Forensic Sciences*, 18, 33–43.

HERDT, G. (1981) *Guardians of the Flutes*, New York, McGraw-Hill.

HERDT, G. (1985) 'A Comment on Cultural Attributes and Fluidity of Bisexuality', *Journal of Homosexuality*, 10, 53–61.

HIRSCH, D. and ENLOW, R.W. (1984) 'The Effects of the Acquired Immune Deficiency Syndrome on Gay Life Styles and the Gay Individual', *Annals of the New York Academy of Sciences*, 437, 273–282.

HORTON, M. and AGGLETON, P. (1989) 'Perverts, Inverts and Experts: The Cultural Production of an AIDS Research Paradigm', in AGGLETON, P., HART, G. and DAVIES, P. (Eds), *AIDS: Social Representations, Social Practices*, Lewes, Falmer Press.

HUNT, A.J., DAVIES, P.M., WEATHERBURN, P., COXON, A.P.M. and McMANUS, T.J. (1991) 'Changes in Sexual Behaviour in a Large Cohort of Homosexual Men in England and Wales', *British Medical Journal*, 302, 505–506.

JOSEPH, J.G., ADIB, S.M., KOOPMAN, J.S. and OSTROW, D.G. (1990) 'Behavioural Change in Longitudinal Studies: Adoption of Condom Use by Homosexual/Bisexual Men', *American Journal of Public Health*, 80, 1513–1514.

JOSEPH, J.G., MONTGOMERY, S., EMMONS, C., KESSLER, R., OSTROW, D., WORTMAN, C., O'BRIEN, D., ELLER, M. and ESHLEMAN, S. (1987a) 'Magnitude and Determinants of Behavioural Risk Reduction: Longitudinal Analysis of a Cohort at Risk for AIDS', *Psychology and Health*, 1, 73–96.

JOSEPH, J.G., MONTGOMERY, S.B., EMMONS, C.A., KIRSCHT, J.P., KESSLER, R.C., OSTROW, D.G., WORTMAN, C.B., O'BRIEN, K., ELLER, M. and ESHLEMAN, S. (1987b) 'Perceived Risk of AIDS: Assessing the Behavioral and Psychological Consequences in a Cohort of Gay Men', *Journal of Applied Social Psychology*, 17, 3, 231–250.

KALDOR, J., WILLIAMSON, P., GOLD, J., GRIMM, P., GUINAN, J., LEARMONT, J., TINDALL, B. and COOPER, D.A. (1991) 'Sero-conversion in Sydney: Measuring the Cutting Edge of the HIV Epidemic', Paper to the Seventh International Conference on AIDS, Florence, 16–21 June.

KINGSLEY, L.A., *et al.* (1987) 'Risk Factors for Seroconversion to Human Immunodeficiency Virus among Male Homosexuals', *The Lancet*, February, 345–348.

KINSEY, A.C., POMEROY, W.B. and MARTIN, C.E. (1948) *Sexual Behavior in the Human Male*, Philadelphia, Pa., Saunders.

KINSEY, A.C., POMEROY, W.B., MARTIN, C.E. and GEBHARD, P.H. (1953) *Sexual Behavior in the Human Female*, Philadelphia, Pa., Saunders.

KINSMAN, G. (1987) *The Regulation of Desire*, Montreal, Black Rose.

KIPPAX, S. and CRAWFORD, J. (in press) 'Flaws in the Theory of Reasoned Action', in TERRY, D.J., GALLOIS, C. and McCAMISH, M.M. (Eds), *The Theory of Reasoned Action: Its Application to AIDS-Preventive Behaviour*, London, Pergamon.

KIPPAX, S., BOND, G., SINNOTT, V., CRAWFORD, J., DOWSETT, G.W., BAXTER, D., BERG, R., CONNELL, R.W. and WATSON, L. (1989) *Social Aspects of the Prevention of AIDS: Study A, Report No. 4. Regional Differences in the Responses of Gay and Bisexual Men to AIDS: The Australian Capital Territory*, Sydney, Macquarie University, School of Behavioural Sciences.

KIPPAX, S., CRAWFORD, J., BOND, G., SINNOTT, V., BAXTER, D., BERG, R., CONNELL, R.W., DOWSETT, G.W. and WATSON, L. (1988) *Social Aspects of the Prevention of AIDS: Study A, Technical Report No. 2. Information about AIDS: The Accuracy of Knowledge Possessed by Gay and Bisexual Men*, Sydney, Macquarie University, School of Behavioural Sciences.

KIPPAX, S., CRAWFORD, J., CONNELL, R.W., DOWSETT, G.W., WATSON, L., RODDEN, P., BAXTER, D. and BERG, R. (1992) 'The Importance of Gay Community in the Prevention of HIV Transmission: A Study of Australian Men Who Have Sex with Men', in AGGLETON, P., DAVIES, P. and HART, G. (Eds), *AIDS: Rights, Risk and Reason*, London, Falmer Press.

KIPPAX, S., CRAWFORD, J., DAVIS, M., RODDEN, P. and DOWSETT, G.W. (1993) 'Sustaining Safe Sex: A Longitudinal Study of a Sample of Homosexual Men', *AIDS*, 7, 2, 257–263.

KIPPAX, S., CRAWFORD, J., DOWSETT, G.W., BOND, G., SINNOTT, V., BAXTER, D., BERG, R., CONNELL, R.W. and WATSON, L. (1990) 'Gay Men's Knowledge of HIV Transmission and "Safe" Sex: A Question of Accuracy', *Australian Journal of Social Issues*, 25, 3, 199–219.

KIPPAX, S., CRAWFORD, J. and WALDBY, C. (1989) 'Epidemiology for the Masses: HIV Prevention Strategies for the Population or the Individual', Paper to the Australian Conference on Medical and Scientific Aspects of AIDS and HIV Infection, Sydney, 30 August.

KIRSCHT, J.P. and JOSEPH, J.G. (1989) 'The Health Belief Model: Some Implications for Behavior Change, with Reference to Homsoexual Males', in MAYS, V.M., ALBEE, G.W. and SCHNEIDER, S.F. (Eds), *Primary Prevention of AIDS: Psychological Approaches*, New York, Sage Publications.

KOTARBA, J.A. and LANG, N.A. (1986) 'Gay Lifestyle Change and AIDS: Preventive Health Care', in FELDMAN, D.A. and JOHNSON, T.M. (Eds), *The Social Dimensions of AIDS*, New York, Praeger.

KRAFFT-EBING (1965) *Psychopathia Sexualis*, New York, Paperback Library (original work published 1886).

LUPTON, D. (1991a) 'AIDS and the Popular Media: A New Perspective at Florence', *AIDS Care*, 3, 4, 447–449.

LUPTON, D. (1991b) 'Apocalypse to Banality: Changes in Metaphors about AIDS in the Australian Press', *Australian Journal of Communication*, 18, 2, 66–74.

McCAMISH, M. (1987) 'Operation Vampire', Paper presented at NACAIDS Seminar, Sydney.

McCUSICK, L., HORSTMAN, W. and COATES, T. (1985) 'AIDS and Sexual Behaviour Reported by Gay Men in San Francisco', *American Journal of Public Health*, 75, 493–496.

MACDONALD, A. (1981) 'Bisexuality: Some Comments on Research and Theory', *Journal of Homosexuality*, 6, 21–36.

MANTELL, J.E. (1989) 'AIDS Health Promotion among New York Males Who Have Sex with Males', Paper to the World Health Organisation Workshop on Health Promotion Activities Directed towards Gay and Bisexual Men, Geneva, 29–31 May.

MARCUSE, H. (1955) *Eros and Civilization*, Boston, Mass., Beacon Press.

MARKOVA, I. and WILKIE, P. (1987) 'Representations, Concepts and Social Change: The Phenomenon of AIDS', *Journal for the Theory of Social Behaviour*, 17, 389–409.

MARSHALL, S. (1990) 'Picturing Deviancy', in BOFFIN, T. and GUPTA, S. (Eds), *Ecstatic Antibodies: Resisting the AIDS Mythology*, London, Rivers Oram Press.

MASTERS, W.H. and JOHNSON, V.E. (1966) *Human Sexual Response*, Boston, Mass., Little and Brown.

MILLAN, G. and ROSS, M. (1987) 'AIDS and Gay Youth: Attitudes and Lifestyle Modifications in Young Male Homosexuals', *Community Health Studies*, 11, 1, 50–53.

NATIONAL CENTRE IN HIV EPIDEMIOLOGY AND CLINICAL RESEARCH [NCHECR] (1992a) *Australian HIV Surveillance Report*, 8 (supplement 3), July.

NATIONAL CENTRE IN HIV EPIDEMIOLOGY AND CLINICAL RESEARCH [NCHECR] (1992b) *National Working Group on HIV Projections of the HIV Epidemic in Australia, 1981–1994*, Sydney, University of New South Wales, NCHECR.

NATIONAL CENTRE IN HIV EPIDEMIOLOGY AND CLINICAL RESEARCH [NCHECR] (1992c) *Australian HIV Surveillance Report*, 8 (supplement 1), January.

NEW SOUTH WALES HEALTH DEPARTMENT (1990) *Report: Planning for HIV/AIDS Care and Treatment Services in New South Wales 1990–1994*, Sydney, State Health Publication (AIDS) 90–68, prepared by the AIDS Bureau.

O'REILLY, C. (1991) *Western Sydney Men Who Have Sex with Men Project: A Report on Initial Outreach Work to Non-Gay Identifying Men Who Have Sex with Men Living in Western Sydney*, Sydney, Western Sydney Area Health Service, AIDS Unit, Education and Training Section.

PARNELL, B. (1992) 'Changing Behaviour', in TIMEWELL, E., *et al.* (Eds), *AIDS in Australia*, Sydney, Prentice-Hall.

PATTON, C. (1989) 'Resistance and the Erotic', in AGGLETON, P., HART, G. and DAVIES, P. (Eds), *AIDS: Social Representations, Social Practices*, London, Falmer Press.

PATTON, C. (1990) *Inventing AIDS*, New York, Routledge.

PAUL, J.P. (1984) 'The Bisexual Identity: An Idea without Social Recognition', *Journal of Homosexuality*, 9, 45–63.

PENNY, R., MARKS, R., BERGER, J., MARRIOT, D. and BRYANT, D. (1983) 'Acquired Immune Deficiency Syndrome', *Medical Journal of Australia*, 13, 554–557.

POLLAK, M. (1989) 'AIDS Prevention Activities and Their Impact on Behaviour: The Case of French Homo- and Bi-sexuals', Paper to the World Health Organisation Workshop on Health Promotion Activities Directed towards Gay and Bisexual Men, Geneva, 29–31 May.

REICHE, R. and DANNECKER, M. (1977) 'Male Homosexuality in West Germany: A Sociological Investigation', *Journal of Sex Research*, 13, 1, pp. 35–53.

RESEARCH AND DECISIONS CORPORATION (1984) *Designing an Effective AIDS Prevention Strategy for San Francisco: Results from the First Probability Sample of an Urban Gay Male Community*, San Francisco, Calif., San Francisco AIDS Foundation.

ROSS, M.W. (1986) *Psychovenereology*, New York, Praeger.

ROSS, M.W. (1988) 'Prevalence of Classes at Risk Behaviours for HIV Infection in a Randomly Selected Australian Population', *Journal of Sex Research*, 25, 441–450.

RUBIN, L.B. (1976) *Worlds of Pain: Life in the Working-class Family*, New York, Basic Books.

SECORD, P.F. (Ed.) (1982) *Explaining Human Behavior*, Beverley Hills, Calif., Sage.

SHERR, L. (1987) 'An Evaluation of the UK Government Health Education Campaign on AIDS', *Psychology and Health*, 1, 1, 61–72.

SHILTS, R. (1988) *And the Band Played On: Politics, People and the AIDS Epidemic*, Harmondsworth, Penguin.

SIEGEL, K., BAUMAN, L.J., CHRIST, G.H. and KROWN, S. (1988) 'Patterns of Change in Sexual Behaviour among Gay Men in New York City', *Archives of Sexual Behavior*, 17, 6, 481–497.

SINNOTT, V. and TODD, S. (1987) 'The VAC Community Education Evaluation Project', Paper presented at NACAIDS seminar, Sydney.

SINNOTT, V. and TODD, S. (1988) *Victorian AIDS Council Community Education Evaluation Project: Final Report*, Melbourne, Victorian AIDS Council.

SOLOMON, P.J., FAZEKAS DE ST GROTH, C. and WILSON, S.R. (1990) 'Use of the Back Projection Method for Predictions of the Australian AIDS Epidemic', in SOLOMON, P.J., *et al.* (Eds), *Projections of Acquired Immune Deficiency Syndrome in Australia Using Data to the End of September 1989*, Canberra, Australian National University, National Centre for Epidemiology and Population Health, Working Papers No. 16, pp. 31–39.

SONTAG, S. (1988) *AIDS and Its Metaphors*, New York, Farrar, Straus and Giroux.

STALL, R. and EKSTRAND, M. (1989) 'Implications of Relapse from Safe Sex', *Focus*, 4, 3.

STALL, R., EKSTRAND, M., POLLACK, L., McCUSICK, L. and COATES, T.J. (1990) 'Relapse from Safer Sex: The Next Challenge for AIDS Prevention Efforts', *Journal of the Acquired Immune Deficiency Syndrome*, 3, 1181–1187.

STRUNIN, L. and HINGSON, R. (1987) 'Acquired Immunodeficiency Syndrome and Adolescents: Knowledge, Beliefs, and Attitudes and Behaviours', *Pediatrics*, 79, 825–828.

SYDNEY AIDS STUDY GROUP (1984) 'The Sydney AIDS Project', *Medical Journal of Australia*, 141, 569–573.

TIELMAN, R.A.P. (1989) 'AIDS Health Promotion Activities in the Netherlands among Men with Homosexual Contacts', Paper to the World Health Organisation Workshop on Health Promotion Activities Directed towards Gay and Bisexual Men, Geneva, 29–31 May.

TINDALL, B., SWANSON, C., DONOVAN, B. and COOPER, D.A. (1989) 'Sexual Practices and Condom Usage in a Cohort of Homosexual Men in Relation to Human Immunodeficiency Virus Status', *Medical Journal of Australia*, 151, 318–322.

TULLOCH, J. (1989) 'Australian Television and the Representation of AIDS', *Australian Journal of Communication*, 16, 101–124.

VAN REYK, P. (1990) *On the Beat: A Report on an Outreach Program of AIDS Preventative Education for Men Who Have Sex with Men*, Sydney, AIDS Council of New South Wales.

WADSWORTH, Y. (1987) 'Values/ideologies in Social Research: The Proof of the Theoretical Pudding Lies in Its Practical Eating', in *Local Knowledge and Local Social Work Practice*, Melbourne, University of Melbourne, Department of Social Work, pp. 52–72.

WATNEY, S. (1987) *Policing Desire: Pornography, AIDS and the Media*, London, Comedia.

WATNEY, S. (1990) 'Safer Sex as Community Practice', in AGGLETON, P., DAVIES, P. and HART, G. (Eds), *AIDS: Individual, Cultural and Policy Dimensions*, London, Falmer Press.

WATTERS, J.K. and BIERNACKI, P. (1989) 'Targeted Sampling: Options for the Study of Hidden Populations', *Social Problems*, 36, 4, 416–430.

WEEKS, J. (1977) *Coming Out: Homosexual Politics in Britain from the Nineteenth Century to the Present*, London, Quartet.

WEEKS, J. (1981) *Sex, Politics and Society: The Regulation of Sexuality since 1800*, London, Longman.

WEEKS, J. (1985) *Sexuality and Its Discontents*, London, Routledge and Kegan Paul.

WEEKS, J. (1986) *Sexuality*, London, Horwood and Tavistock.

WEEKS, J. (1987) 'Questions of identity', in CAPLAN, P. (Ed.), *The Cultural Construction of Sexuality*, London, Tavistock Publications.

WEINSTEIN, N.D. (1984) 'Why It Won't Happen to Me: Perceptions of Risk Factors and Illness Susceptibility', *Health Psychology*, 3, 431–457.

WILLIAM, D.C. (1984) 'The Prevention of AIDS by Modifying Sexual Behaviour', *Annals of the New York Academy of Sciences*, 437, 283–285.

WILLIAMS, L.S. (1986) 'AIDS Risk Reduction: A Community Health Education Intervention for Minority High Risk Group Members', *Health Education Quarterly*, 13, 4, 407–421.

WILLIAMS, W.L. (1986) *The Spirit and the Flesh: Sexual Diversity in the American Indian Culture*, Boston, Mass., Beacon Press.

WILLIS, E. (1983) *Medical Dominance*, Sydney, Allen and Unwin.

WINKELSTEIN, W., SAMUEL, M., PADIAN, N.S., WILEY, J.A., LANG, W., ANDERSON, R.E. and LEVY, J.A. (1987) 'The San Francisco Men's Health Study: III. Reduction in Human Immunodeficiency Virus Transmission among Homosexual/Bisexual Men, 1982–86', *American Journal of Public Health*, 76, 685–689.

ZINIK, G. (1985) 'Identity Conflict or Adaptive Flexibility? Bisexuality Reconsidered', *Journal of Homosexuality*, 11, 7–19.

Appendix 1:
SAPA Project Publications

SAPA Monograph Series

We have followed the convention that the person/s primarily responsible for the paper are listed first; the others follow usually in alphabetical order.

1 Connell, R.W.,Crawford, J., Kippax, S., Dowsett, G.W., Bond, G., Baxter, D., Berg, R. and Watson, L. (1987) *Method and Sample.*

2 Kippax, S., Crawford, J., Bond, G., Sinnott, V., Baxter, D., Berg, R., Connell, R.W., Dowsett, G.W. and Watson, L. (1988) *Information about AIDS: The Accuracy of Knowledge Possessed by Gay and Bisexual Men.*

3 Connell, R.W., Crawford, J., Bond, G., Sinnott, V., Baxter, D., Berg, R., Dowsett, G., Kippax, S. and Watson, L. (1988) *Facing the Epidemic: Changes in the Sexual and Social Lives of Gay and Bisexual Men in Response to the AIDS Crisis, and Their Implications for AIDS Prevention Strategies.*

4 Kippax, S., Bond, G., Sinnott, V., Crawford, J., Dowsett, G.W., Baxter, D., Berg, R., Connell, R.W. and Watson, L. (1989) *Regional Differences in the Responses of Gay and Bisexual Men to AIDS: The Australian Capital Territory.*

5 Connell, R.W. and Kippax, S. (1989) *Practice and Pleasure: Sexuality in a Sample of Gay and Bisexual Men.*

6   Connell, R.W., Crawford, J., Dowsett, G.W., Kippax, S., Sinnott, V., Rodden, P., Baxter, D., Berg, R. and Watson, L. (1989) *Unsafe Anal Practice among Homosexual and Bisexual Men.*

7   Kippax, S., Crawford, J., Connell, R.W., Watson, L., Dowsett, G.W., Rodden, P., Baxter, D. and Berg, R. (1990) *The Role of Gay Community in the Prevention of HIV Transmission.*

8   Crawford, J., Dowsett, G.W., Kippax, S., Connell, R.W., Baxter, D., Berg, R. and Watson, L. (1992) *Gay and Bisexual: Bisexual and Gay. The Sexual Behaviour of Men Who Have Sex with Men and Women in an Australian Sample of Gay and Bisexual Men.*

Technical Reports

1   Dowsett, G.W., Connell, R.W., Crawford, J., Kippax, S., Rodden, P., Sinnott, V., Baxter, D. and Watson, L. (1987) 'Frequency Tabulations for Selected Items'.

2   Sinnott, V., Connell, R.W., Crawford, J., Dowsett, G.W., Kippax, S., Rodden, P., Baxter, D. and Watson, L. (1988) 'A Statistical Report on the Development of Scales'.

3   Dowsett, G.W., Connell, R.W., Crawford, J., Kippax, S., Rodden, P., Sinnott, V., Baxter, D. and Watson, L. (1988) 'Raw Frequencies on Condom Use in a Sample of Gay and Bisexual Men'.

4   Dowsett, G.W., Connell, R.W., Crawford, J., Kippax, S., Rodden, P., Sinnott, V., Baxter, D. and Watson, L. (1989) 'Oral-genital Sex in a Sample of Gay and Bisexual Men'.

5   Dowsett, G.W., Connell, R.W., Crawford, J., Kippax, S., Rodden, P., Sinnott, V., Baxter, D. and Watson, L. (1989) 'Sexual Practices with Regular and Casual Partners in a Sample of Gay and Bisexual Men'.

6   Dowsett, G.W., Connell, R.W., Crawford, J., Kippax, S., Rodden, P., Sinnott, V., Baxter, D. and Watson, L. (1989) 'The Effect of Region on AIDS Education and Sexual Behaviour Change among Gay and Bisexual Men'.

7   Rodden, P., Connell, R.W., Crawford, J., Dowsett, G.W., Kippax, S., Sinnott, V., Baxter, D. and Watson, L. (1990) 'Characteristics of Scales: Second Report'.

8   Kippax, S., Dowsett, G.W., Davis, M., Rodden, P. and Crawford, J. (1991) 'Social Aspects of the Prevention of AIDS, 1991 Sustaining Safe Sex Survey' (Technical Report to the Australian Federation of AIDS Organizations and the AIDS Council of NSW).

Further information on the availability of SAPA project publications can be obtained from:

The SAPA Project
School of Behavioural Sciences
Macquarie University
Sydney
New South Wales 2109
Australia

Appendix 2: Description of Sample, Comparison with 1986 Census and VAC Data

Table A2.1. Region

Region	Percentage
Sydney	
Oxford Street quarter	16
Inner city	26
Eastern suburbs	15
Northern suburbs	8
Southern suburbs	3
West and southwestern suburbs	11
Extra-metropolitan NSW	14
Australian Capital Territory	8

Source: SAPA Report No. 1.

Table A2.2. Age

Age	SAPA sample	Males 15+ NSW and ACT	VAC sample
		(percentages)	
<20	4	11	6
20–29	37	22	46
30–39	39	21	28
40–49	14	16	15
50+	5	31	4

Sources: SAPA Report No. 1; 1986 Census Data; Sinnott and Todd (1988).

Table A2.3. Ethnicity

Country of birth	SAPA sample	Males 15+ NSW and ACT	VAC sample
		(percentages)	
Australia and New Zealand	82	73	79
Other English-speaking countries	10	9	10
Europe (excluding UK, Eire)	4	9	7
Asia, Africa, Latin America	3	9	4

Sources: SAPA Report No. 1; 1986 Census Data; Sinnott and Todd (1988).

Table A2.4. Income

Income	SAPA sample	Males 15+ NSW and ACT	Male employees NSW, May 1986
		(percentages)	
<$6000	13	23	4
6001–12,000	8	15	8
12,001–18,000	19	20	20
18,001–26,000	27	20	37
26,001+	32	17	31
NR/DK/not stated	2	5	—

Note: This breakdown of income was unavailable for the Victorian data; the mean income was $23,192 compared to $22,098 in SAPA.
Sources: SAPA Report No. 1; 1986 Census Data; Australian Bureau of Statistics Publication No. 6306.0; Sinnott and Todd (1988).

Table A2.5. Labour Force Status

Status	SAPA sample	Estimated labour force NSW Males 15+ November 1986	VAC sample
		(percentages)	
Not in labour force	9	25	7
Unemployed	8	8	9
Part-time employment	11	4	7
Full-time employment	72	64	76

Sources: SAPA Report No. 1; Australian Bureau of Statistics Publication No. 6201.1; Sinnott and Todd (1988).

Appendix 2

Table A2.6. Occupation

Occupation	SAPA sample: full-time employment (either employee or self-employed)	Males 15+ NSW and ACT
	(percentages)	
Managers and administrators	13	14
Professionals	34	13
Paraprofessionals	9	6
Tradespersons	7	22
Clerks	20	8
Sales workers	11	8
Plant and machine operators	2	11
Labourers n.e.c.	3	15
Other	—	2

Note: These data were not available for the VAC sample.
Sources: SAPA Report No. 1; 1986 Census Data.

Table A2.7. Highest Level of Education

Educational level	Percentage
SAPA sample	
Primary or up to three years high	8
School Certificate (or equivalent)	14
Completed secondary	25
Diploma, trade certificate	13
University or CAE	40
1986 Census	
Not qualified	53
Diploma, trade	21
Degree or higher	9
Other qualification	11
Not stated	9
VAC sample	
Up to School Certificate	23
Forms 5, 6	35
Post-secondary	42

Sources: SAPA Report No. 1; 1986 Census Data; Sinnott and Todd (1988).

Table A2.8. Type of Secondary School

Type of secondary school	SAPA sample	Total secondary enrolments, national	
		(percentages)	
		1967	1983
Public	66	74	72
Catholic, systemic	7	17	19
Catholic, independent	12		
Independent	14	8	9

Note: These data were not available for the VAC sample.
Sources: SAPA Report No. 1; Australian Bureau of Statistics Publication No. 4101.0.

Table A2.9. Religion

Religion	SAPA sample	NSW and ACT males All ages
		(percentages)
Protestant (including Church of England)	27	39
Catholic	16	28
Other denominations or religions	11	11
Agnostic, no religion, NR	46	23

Note: These data were not available for the VAC sample.
Sources: SAPA Report No. 1; 1986 Census Data.

Table A2.10. Household Size

Number of occupants	SAPA sample	Persons, NSW and ACT 1986 Census	VAC sample
		(percentages)	
1	24	7	35
2	44	20	35
3	16	17	16
4–5	12	41	13
6+	3	15	2

Sources: SAPA Report No. 1; 1986 Census Data; Sinnott and Todd (1988).

Table A2.11. Relationships among Variables

	Income	Occupation	Education	Household size
Age	.38	.08	.13	−.33
Income		.28	.34	−.19
Occupation			−.15	−.02
Education level				−.06

Source: SAPA Report No. 1.

Appendix 3: Definition of Regions

Region in sample division	Postcodes	ABS statistical subdivision (SSD)
Oxford Street environs	2010,2011 2012	Inner Sydney SSD
Inner city	all others within:	Inner Sydney SSD
Eastern suburbs		Eastern Suburbs SSD
Northern suburbs		Lower Northern Sydney, Manly-Warringah, Hornsby-Kuring-gai SSDs
Southern suburbs		St George-Sutherland SSD
West and southwestern suburbs		Inner Western Sydney, Central Western Sydney, Canterbury-Bankstown, Blacktown-Baulkham Hills, Fairfield-Liverpool, Outer Western Sydney, Outer South-Western Sydney SSDs
Extra-metropolitan NSW		Hunter, Richmond-Tweed, Northern, Illawarra, Central Western, North Western SSDs
Australian Capital Territory	2600–2617 2902–2906	

Note: There were two cases in the sample whose permanent residence was in other states.

Appendix 4: Additional Information about Sexuality Data

Table A4.1. *Mode in Sexuality*

Section of experience/enjoyment item intercorrelation matrix showing clear mode effect for anal but not oral-genital sex. I = insertive, R = receptive. Brackets mark coefficients for different modes of the same practice. Asterisks mark coefficients for the same mode of similar practices. (See discussion in text.)

		Oral-genital sex				Anal intercourse					
		No ejaculation		With ejaculation		No condom		Withdrawal		With condom	
		I	R	I	R	I	R	I	R	I	R
Oral-genital											
No ejaculation	I	1.00	(.46)	.26*	.11	.10	.09	.33	.23	.19	.17
	R		1.00	.23	.16*	.14	.14	.28	.29	.15	.12
With ejaculation	I			1.00	(.42)	.31	.17	.13	.07	.13	.10
	R				1.00	.20	.23	.15	.17	.04	.13
Anal intercourse											
No condom	I					1.00	(.35)	.39*	.20	.38*	.24
	R						1.00	.14	.58*	.17	.61*
Withdrawal	I							1.00	(.50)	.28*	.19
	R								1.00	.19	.52*
With condom	I									1.00	(.53)
	R										1.00

Source: Connell and Kippax (1990).

Appendix 4

Table A4.2. Bivariate Relationships of Three Sexual Practice Scales

Probability levels shown are for F test in analysis of variance using categories shown, except for final five rows which are probability levels for correlation coefficients. *p < .05, **p < .01, ***p < .001.

	Practice scales means		
	OTP	EAP	IEP
STRUCTURE VARIABLES			
Age			
<20 (n = 22)	4.95	2.95	0.45
20–29 (n = 200)	5.38	3.73	0.55
30–39 (n = 208)	5.41	3.77	0.98
40–49 (n = 77)	5.36	3.45	0.87
50+ (n = 28)	4.92	3.71	0.61
Region			
Oxford Street neighbourhood (84)	5.48	4.25	1.21
Inner city (138)	5.40	3.60	0.78
Eastern suburbs (82)	5.24	3.43	0.58
Northern suburbs (43)	5.67	3.88	0.74
Southern suburbs (14)	5.43	3.21	0.64
West and Southwestern suburbs (57)	5.16	3.65	0.60
Extra-metropolitan NSW (75)	5.16	3.52	0.64
Australian Capital Territory (42)	5.36	3.50	0.62
Country of birth			
Australia and New Zealand (439)	5.34	3.67	0.82
Other English-speaking (54)	5.50	4.13	0.63
Non-English-speaking (39)	5.36	3.10	0.23
Religion			
Protestant (144)	5.42	4.00	1.04
Catholic (88)	5.28	3.39	0.63
Other religions (57)	5.19	3.72	0.49
Agnostic/none (241)	5.36	3.55	0.70
Labour force status			
Employee, full-time (323)	5.45	3.98	0.75
Self-employed, full-time (60)	5.23	3.81	1.05
Part-time work (60)	5.32	3.33	0.70
Not in workforce (48)	5.06	3.21	0.65
Unemployed (41)	5.17	3.32	0.59
Occupation			
Managers/professionals (184)	5.52	3.75	0.78
Paraprofessionals/clerks (113)	5.39	3.73	0.71
Sales/manual (91)	5.35	4.10	0.89
Annual income			
<$12,000 (113)	5.13	3.19	0.56
$12,001–18,000 (100)	5.22	3.70	0.64
$18,000–26,000 (142)	5.46	3.74	0.97

Table A4.2.   (Cont.)

	Practice scale means		
	OTP	EAP	IEP
Highest level of education			
Up to Year 10 (115)	5.05	3.70	0.60
Completed high school (134)	5.54	4.04	0.99
Diploma or trade certificate (71)	5.34	3.46	0.58
Some college of university (213)	5.39	3.49	0.77
MILIEU VARIABLES			
Relationship status			
None at present (64)	3.62	1.93	0.30
Monogamous (112)	5.61	4.07	0.65
Several at same time (35)	5.86	5.14	1.60
Regular relationship plus casual sex (151)	5.70	4.25	1.15
Casual only (165)	5.54	3.35	0.50
		**	**
Household size			
One person (129)	5.21	3.30	0.66
Two people (237)	5.49	3.80	0.88
Three people (83)	5.34	3.99	0.90
Four or more (81)	5.14	3.57	0.41
Own sexual identity			
Gay/camp/homosexual (348)	5.36	3.69	0.85
Bisexual (40)	5.53	3.81	0.75
Other/heterosexual (15)	3.87	2.67	0.93
Attributed sexual identity			
Gay/camp/homosexual (348)	5.36	3.69	0.85
Bisexual (32)	5.53	3.81	0.75
Heterosexual (93)	5.38	3.67	0.55
Unsure/don't know (57)	5.10	3.70	0.51
Use any drugs for relaxation and pleasure (includes alcohol and tobacco)			
Yes (470)	5.38	3.75	0.80
No (65)	5.09	3.25	0.49
Importance of anal intercourse			
Very important (112)	5.30	4.29	1.04
Quite important (204)	5.40	4.05	0.82
Not important (166)	5.34	3.40	0.61
No response/don't know (53)	5.26	1.79	0.40
		**	*
CORRELATION WITH PRACTICE SCALES			
	OTP	EAP	IEP
MILIEU VARIABLES (SCALES)			
Gay community involvement (GCI)	0.06	0.05	0.14**
Social engagement (SCE)	0.15**	0.16	0.13**
Sexual engagement (SXE)	0.24**	0.24**	0.24**
Gay identity disclosure (GID)	−0.02	0.04	0.13**

Table A4.2. (Cont.)

	Practice scale means		
	OTP	EAP	IEP
SITUATION VARIABLES			
How many friends practise safe sex			
All (36)	5.42	3.44	0.47
Most (287)	5.46	3.67	0.86
A few (42)	5.29	4.14	0.43
None/don't know (32)	5.25	2.62	0.13
			*
Feelings about condoms			
Completely acceptable (167)	5.37	3.46	0.66
Quite acceptable (297)	5.35	3.75	0.80
Quite unacceptable (53)	5.45	4.15	0.89
Completely unacceptable (9)	4.56	4.00	1.22
Pursues AIDS information in media			
Yes (499)	5.35	3.65	0.75
No (35)	5.46	4.00	1.00
Antibody test status			
No test/no response (174)	5.25	2.83	0.39
Negative (270)	5.42	3.86	0.69
Positive (91)	5.32	4.73	1.69
		**	**
CORRELATION WITH PRACTICE SCALES			
	OTP	EAP	IEP
SITUATION VARIABLES (SCALES)			
AIDS pamphlet awareness (PA)[a]	0.03	0.09*	0.07
Knowledge about safe sex (KSS)[b]	0.09*	0.07	0.01
Knowledge about unsafe sex (KUS)[c]	−0.06	−0.07*	−0.02
General Issues[d]	−0.10**	0.04	0.03
Contact with epidemic (CE)[e]	0.03	0.09*	0.15**

Notes: a High scores mean respondent recognizes more of the AIDS pamphlets circulating at time.
     b High scores reflect correct (by AIDS educators' standards) judgments about practices that are in fact safe.
     c High scores reflect correct (by AIDS educators' standards) judgments about practices that are in fact unsafe.
     d High scores reflect rash or optimistic judgment about AIDS issues in general, e.g., immunity, early availability of a vaccine.
     e High scores reflect personal links with people with AIDS.
Source: Connell and Kippax (1990).

Table A4.3. *Bivariate Relationships of 'Danger' in Anal Practice*

'Danger' measure is whether had unprotected anal intercourse (insertive, receptive or both) in the last six months. This is examined separately for respondents with regular partners and with casual (these groups overlap). Significance tested by chi-squared in cross-classifications, and by F test in analysis of variance for scales. Probability levels less than 0.1 are shown.

	Those with regular partners				Those with casual partners			
	High danger (either or both modes) %	Low danger (neither mode) %	n	p	High danger (either or both modes) %	Low danger (neither mode) %	n	p
STRUCTURE VARIABLES								
Age								
Less than 25	43	57	7		42	5	19	
25–29	49	51	118		30	70	139	
30–39	50	50	117		31	69	156	
More than 39	71	29	56	.05	33	67	80	ns
Region								
Oxford Street	49	51	53		32	68	63	
Inner city	42	58	78		23	77	103	
Eastern suburbs	56	44	45		28	72	61	
Northern suburbs	55	45	22		32	68	34	
Southern suburbs	71	29	7		50	50	8	
West and Southwestern suburbs	63	37	32		49	51	41	
Extra-metropolitan NSW	68	32	38		34	66	53	
Australian Capital Territory	57	43	23	ns	36	65	31	ns
Country of birth								
Australia/New Zealand	52	48	240		33	67	317	
Other English-speaking	61	39	36		27	73	44	
Non-English-speaking	57	43	21	ns	23	77	30	ns

Table A4.3. (Cont.)

	Those with regular partners				Those with casual partners			
	High danger (either or both modes) %	Low danger (neither mode) %	n	p	High danger (either or both modes) %	Low danger (neither mode) %	n	p
Religion								ns
Protestant	69	31	88		35	65	317	
Catholic	44	56	45		35	65	68	
Other religions	48	52	27		34	73	41	
Agnostic/none	49	51	136		27	73	179	
Labour force status				.007				ns
Employee, full-time	56	44	185		35	65	102	
Self-employed, full-time	54	46	37		22	78	45	
Part-time work	42	58	36		20	80	45	
Not in workforce	55	45	20		37	63	35	
Unemployed	53	47	19		38	62	32	
Occupation (full-time workers)				ns				.04
Managers/professionals	50	50	113		24	76	135	
Paraprofessionals/clerks	60	40	58		37	63	82	
Sales/manual	57	43	56		40	60	70	
Annual income				ns				ns
Less than $12,000	52	48	52		28	72	88	
$12,001–$18,000	55	45	58		30	70	71	
$18,001–$26,000	54	46	74		34	66	98	
$26,001 and above	56	44	108		32	68	128	

Highest level of education				ns				ns
Up to Year 10	63	37	48		41	59	85	
Completed high school	54	46	81		30	70	100	
Diploma or trade certificate	51	49	45		36	64	50	
Some college or university	50	50	122		27	73	158	
MILIEU VARIABLES								
Current sexual relationship status				.03				ns
None at present	50	50	8		32	68	44	
Monogamous	65	35	109		21	79	19	
Several at same time	52	48	33		40	60	30	
Regular relationship plus casual sex	47	53	140		26	74	138	
Casual sex only	25	75	8		36	64	162	
Own sexual identity				ns				ns
Homosexual/gay	55	45	277		30	70	345	
Bisexual	36	64	14		40	60	35	
Other	33	67	3		36	64	11	
Attributed sexual identity				ns				ns
Gay/homosexual	52	48	205		30	70	258	
Bisexual	36	64	14		40	60	35	
Straight, heterosexual	61	39	46		43	57	63	
Unsure, don't know	65	35	31		26	74	39	

Table A4.3. (Cont.)

	Those with regular partners				Those with casual partners			
	High danger (either or both modes) %	Low danger (neither mode) %	n	p	High danger (either or both modes) %	Low danger (neither mode) %	n	p
Use any drugs for relaxation and pleasure (includes alcohol and tobacco)								
Yes	52	48	266		31	69	347	
No	66	34	32	ns	38	62	47	ns
MILIEU SCALES OF ATTACHMENT	n = 160	n = 138			n = 125	n = 269		
Sexual Engagement (SXE)								
Mean:	23.9	25.3		.01	27.9	26.3		.0001
SD:	4.8	4.5			4.1	3.4		
Social Engagement (SCE)								
Mean:	19.2	19.6		.09	18.6	19.2		.03
SD:	2.0	2.1			2.9	2.3		
Gay Community Involvement (GCI)	n = 144	n = 126			n = 115	n = 235		
Mean:	32.8	33.3		ns	31.6	33.2		.007
SD:	5.1	5.0			5.3	5.3		
Gay Identity Disclosure (GID)								
Mean:	4.4	4.4		ns	3.9	4.3		.04
SD:	1.9	1.7			2.1	1.9		

SITUATION VARIABLES

	%	%	n	p	%	%	n	p
How many friends practise safe sex								
All	32	68	25		11	89	26	
Most	50	50	155		24	76	222	
Some	61	39	79		44	56	92	
A few/none	72	28	25		67	33	27	
Don't know	73	27	11	.06	32	68	22	.0000
Making point of reading articles, hearing programs about AIDS								
Yes	52	48	276		31	69	368	
No	73	27	22	.06	42	58	26	ns
Antibody test status								
No test/no response	48	52	83		35	65	130	
Positive	46	54	56		29	71	68	
Negative	59	41	159	30 ns	70	30	196	ns

Table A4.3. (Cont.)

SCALES RELATING TO SITUATION

		n = 160	n = 138	P	n = 125	n =269	P
AIDS Pamphlet Awareness (PA)	Mean: SD:	4.3 2.1	4.8 2.1	0.3	4.0 2.1	4.4 2.2	0.5
Knowledge about Safe Sex (KSS)	Mean: SD:	7.0 3.3	7.5 3.4	ns	7.0 3.2	7.2 3.4	ns
Knowledge about Unsafe Sex (KUS)	Mean: SD:	6.5 2.3	6.8 2.2	ns	6.1 2.2	7.0 2.1	.0001
General Issues (GI)	Mean: SD:	24.8 3.7	26.1 3.7	.003	24.1 4.1	25.5 3.7	.0006
Contact with Epidemic (CE)	Mean: SD:	1.5 1.0	1.7 1.0	.07	1.2 1.1	1.6 1.1	.003

Source: Connell at al., (1990).

Appendix 5: Descriptions of Scales Developed from the Questionnaire Responses

Knowledge of Social Practices (KSP)

With regard to passing on the AIDS virus, how safe or risky are these forms of social contact?

Hugging
Shaking hands
Sharing a joint
Kissing with closed mouth
Sharing a bath
Sharing a towel
Sharing a toothbrush[a]
Sharing a razor[a]
Sharing a swimming pool
Sharing a glass or spoon
Using public toilets
Using public telephones

Scoring:

All items except those marked[a] scored 1 if the response was very safe, otherwise 0.

[a] Items scored 1 if the response was 'small risk', otherwise 0.

Characteristics of scale:

Number of items	12
Cronbach's alpha	.68
Range	0–12
Mean	9.9
Standard deviation	1.93
High score	High knowledge of safety of social practices
Low score	Low knowledge of safety of social practices

Knowledge of Unsafe Sexual Practices (KUS)

With respect to passing on the AIDS virus, how safe or unsafe do you think each of the sexual activities listed below is (whether you have tried them or not)?

Rimming (giving)[a]
Being rimmed (receiving)[a]
Fucking without condoms (insertive)[b]
Fucking without condoms (receptive)[b]
Fucking without coming (insertive)[c]
Fucking without coming (receptive)[c]
Sucking and swallowing semen[b]
Being sucked and ejaculating[b]
Fisting partner[a]
Being fisted[a]

Scoring:

[a] Scored 1 if response was 'small risk' or 'not at all safe', otherwise 0.
[b] Scored 1 if response was 'not at all safe', otherwise 0.
[c] Scored 1 if response was 'small risk', otherwise 0.

Characteristics of scale:

Number of items	10
Cronbach's alpha	.70
Range	0–10

Mean	6.68
Standard deviation	2.23
High score	High Knowledge of unsafe sex
Low score	Low Knowledge of unsafe sex

Knowledge of Safe Sex Practices (KSS)

With respect to passing on the AIDS virus, how safe or unsafe do you think each of the sexual activities listed below is (whether you have tried them or not)?

Wet/deep kissing
Dry kissing
Fucking with condom (insertive)
Fucking with condom (receptive)
Sucking and not swallowing semen
Being sucked and not ejaculating
Mutual masturbation
Watersports — in mouth (receptive)
Watersports — in mouth (insertive)
Being urinated on
Urinating on your partner
Finger fucking (insertive)
Finger fucking (receptive)
Sensuous touching
SM dominance without blood

Scoring:

All items scored 1 if response was 'very safe', otherwise 0.

Scale characteristics:

Number of items	15
Cronbach's alpha	.80
Range	0–15 (13 highest score)
Mean	7.10
Standard deviation	3.29

High score	High knowledge of safe sex practices
Low score	Low knowledge of safe sex practices

Pamphlet Awareness (PA)

Which of the following have you seen?

Rubba Me
If Your AIDS Test Proves Positive
When a Friend Has AIDS
Ankali
You'll Never Forget the Feeling
Brad and Steve
Albion Street pamphlet
'Reader's Digest'

Scoring:

All items scored 1 if response was 'yes', otherwise 0.

Characteristics of scale:

Number of items:	9
Cronbach's alpha	.70
Range	0–9
Mean	4.3
Standard deviation	2.2
High score	Sees lots of brochures
Low score	Sees few/no brochures

Adopting Safe Sex (AS)

Has your awareness of AIDS led you to make any changes in your sexual activities?

Yes —	continue
No	
DK/NR	

Which changes:

>> Masturbating alone
>> Reading/watching porn
>> Using condoms
>> Mutual masturbation
>> Sensuous touching
>> 'Safe sex' with regular partner

Scoring:

All items scored as follows:

Response	Score
Stopped	1
Doing it less	2
Never done/about the same/no response	3
Started or doing it more	4

Characteristics of scale:

Number of items	7
Cronbach's alpha	.65
Range	7–28
Mean	23.8
Standard deviation	2.1
High score	Most changes towards safe sex
Low score	Least changes towards safe sex

Relationship Change (RC)

For you, has awareness of AIDS led you to make any changes to your sexual relations?

Cutting down on sex generally
Avoid sex with certain individuals

Avoid sex with antibody negative people
Changing the sort of men I pick up
Changing places I pick men up
Avoid sex with prostitutes
Reduce number of sex partners
Becoming monogamous
Asking partner to become monogamous
Avoid sex with antibody positive people
Avoid sex with people whose antibody status is not known

Scoring:

All items scored 1 if the response was 'Yes', otherwise 0.

Characteristics of scale:

Number of items	11
Cronbach's alpha	.79
Range	0–11
Mean	3.4
Standard deviation	2.7
High score	More relationship changes
Low score	Little/no relationship changes

Oral-Tactile Practices (OTP)

Wet kissing/deep kissing
Dry kissing
Sucking (oral-genital)*
Being sucked (oral-genital)*
Masturbating (jerking off) together
Sensuous touching

* Either with or without ejaculation

Scoring:

All items scored 1 if practice engaged in occasionally or often during the past six months, with either a regular partner, a casual partner, or both regular and casual partners; otherwise 0.

Characteristics of scale:

Number of items	6
Cronbach's alpha	.86
Range	0–6
Mean	5.3
Standard deviation	1.4
High score	Engages in many oral-tactile practices
Low score	Engages in fewer oral-tactile practices

Essentially Anal Practices (EAP)

Oral-anal contact (rimming/roseleafing your partner) (giving)

Oral-anal contact (being rimmed/roseleafed) (receiving)

Anal intercourse (fucking): active-giving (fucking partner and coming inside)*

Anal intercourse (fucking): receiving (being fucked with partner coming)*

Anal intercourse (fucking): without ejaculation (coming): active-giving (fucking partner without coming inside)

Anal intercourse (fucking): without ejaculation (coming): receiving (being fucked without partner coming)

Finger in partner's rectum (finger fucking)

Finger in your rectum (being finger fucked)

* Either with or without condom.

Scoring:

All items scored 1 if practice engaged in occasionally or often during the past six months, with either a regular partner, a casual partner, or both regular and casual partners; otherwise 0.

Characteristics of scale:

Number of items	6
Cronbach's alpha	.79
Range	0–6
Mean	3.7
Standard deviation	2.5
High score	Engages in many anal practices
Low score	Engages in few anal practices

Infrequent Esoteric Practices (IEP)

Having your partner urinate on you (watersports)
Urinating on your partner
Fisting partner (hand/fist in partner's rectum)
Being fisted (hand/fist in your rectum)
Receiving dildo/vibrator/toy
Giving dildo/vibrator/toy
S/M dominance/bondage: giving (top)*
S/M dominance/bondage: receiving (bottom)*

* Either with or without blood.

Scoring:

All items scored 1 if practice engaged in occasionally or often during the past six months, with either a regular partner, a casual partner, or both regular and casual partners; otherwise 0.

Characteristics of scale:

Number of items	8
Cronbach's alpha	.81
Range	0–8
Mean	0.8
Standard deviation	1.5
High score	Engages in many esoteric practices
Low score	Engages in few esoteric practices

General Issues (GI)

I want you to read the following general statements with me and tell me for each one whether you strongly agree, agree, disagree or strongly disagree.

It is unlikely that there will soon be a cure for AIDS[a]
AIDS can be transmitted in *one* sexual contact[a]
Women can't get AIDS through sexual contact[b]
Only people with positive antibody results need to be careful about their sexual activities[b]
People can become immune to AIDS[b]
Someone could pass on AIDS while appearing very healthy[a]
There will soon be a vaccine to prevent AIDS[b]
AIDS is caused by repeated contact with sexually transmitted diseases which wears down the immune system[b]

Scoring:

	Response	Score
a	Strongly agree	1
	Agree	2
	Disagree	4
	Strongly disagree	5
	NR/don't know	3
b	Strongly agree	5
	Agree	4
	Disagree	2
	Strongly disagree	1
	NR/don't know	3

Characteristics of scale:

Number of items	8
Cronbach's alpha	.63
Range	8–40(highest score 28)
Mean	15.0
Standard deviation	3.9
High score	Rash, incautious
Low score	Caution, prudence

Contact with the Epidemic (CE)

Do you know anyone who has AIDS?[a]

Do you know anyone who has died from AIDS?[b]

Have you been involved with the care or nursing of people with AIDS?[b]

Scoring:

	Response	Score
a	No one	0
	Sexual partner,	
	past sexual partner	
	friend/relative	
	acquaintance	1
	NR/don't know	0
b	Yes	1
	No, NR, DK	0

Characteristics of scale:

Number of items	3
Cronbach's alpha	.61
Range	0–3
Mean	1.4
Standard deviation	1.1
High score	High contact with the epidemic
Low score	No/little contact with the epidemic

Sexual Engagement (SXE)

When you're out with your gay friends, where do you usually go?

Saunas[a]
Beats[a]
Sex cinemas[a]
The wall/parlours (i.e., prostitutes)[a]

If you are looking for a sexual partner, where do you go?

> Bars[a]
> Saunas[a]
> Discos/dances[a]
> Private parties/through friends[a]
> Beats[a]
> Bookshops[a]
> Sex cinemas[a]
> The wall/parlours (i.e., prostitutes)[a]
> Gym[a]
> Pool/beach[a]

Do you watch gay porn videos?[b]

How often in the last six months have you done any of the activities below with your regular male partner/s?

> Sex in particular places/venues[b]

How many men have you had sex with in the past six months?[c]

In the past month, how often did you have sex with casual male partners?[d]

How often in the last six months have you done any of the activities below with your casual male partner/s?

> Sex in particular places/venues[b]

Scoring:

	Response	Score
a	Yes	2
	No, NR	1
b	Often	3
	Sometimes	2
	No, never	1
	NR	1
c	None/NR	0
	1	1
	2–10	2

11–50	3
51–200	4
>200	4
None/NR/DK	0
1–5	1
6–15	2
16–30	3
>30	3

d

Characteristics of scale:

Number of items	19
Cronbach's alpha	.79
Range	17–44 (40 highest score)
Mean	25.2
Standard deviation	4.5
High score	High sexual engagement
Low score	Low sexual engagement

Social Engagement (SCE)

How much of your free time do you spend with gay/camp/homosexual men?[a]

How many of your friends are gay/camp/homosexual men?[b]

Do you go out with gay/bisexual friends?[c]

When you're out with your gay friends, where do you usually go?

(Go through list)
Bars[c]
Theatre/concerts/cinema[c]
Discos/dances[c]
Private parties[c]
Bookshops[c]
Pool/beach[c]
Meetings/organizations[c]

Scoring:

	Response	Score
a	None/NR/DK	1
	A little	2
	Some	3
	A lot	4
b	None, a few	0
	Unsure/NR/DK	
	Some	1
	Most	2
	All	3
c	Yes	2
	No/NR/DK	1

Characteristics of scale:

Number of items	10
Cronbach's alpha	.71
Range	9–23
Mean	19.0
Standard deviation	2.5
High score	High social engagement
Low score	Low social engagement

Gay Community Involvement (GCI)

Do you go to any of the following gay community functions?

> Gay sporting groups[a]
> Gay political groups[a]
> Gay social groups[a]
> Gay religious groups[a]
> Gay counselling groups[a]
> AIDS-related groups[a]
> Gay university/college groups[a]

Do you see yourself, personally, as being part of the gay community?[b]

Are you or have you been a member of any gay/bisexual organizations?[a]

Which gay/bisexual organizations are you or have you been a member of ?

> Gay sporting groups[a]
> Gay political groups[a]
> Gay social groups[a]
> Gay religious groups[a]
> Gay counselling groups[a]
> Gay university/college groups[a]

Do you make a point of seeing plays or films with gay themes?[c]

Do you make a point of reading books with gay themes?[c]

Do you make a point of going to gay shops and businesses?[c]

Which gay newspapers/magazines do you read most often?[d]

Do you usually go to a gay-identified doctor?[c]

Scoring:

	Response	Score
a	Yes	2
	No/NR	1
b	Yes	3
	Unsure/DK	2
	No	1
c	Often	3
	Sometimes	2
	Never, no, NR/DK	1
d	None/NR/DK	0
	Mention of one gay magazine	1
	Mention of two	2
	Mention three or more	3

Characteristics of scale:

Number of items	21
Cronbach's alpha	.81

Range	20–48
Mean	32.6
Standard deviation	5.2
High score	High involvement
Low score	Low involvement

Gay Identity Disclosure (GID)

Whom have you told that you are gay/camp/homosexual/bisexual?

Mother[a]
Father[a]
Other relatives
Any straight friends
Any workmates
Any neighbours
Anyone else

Scoring:

Scored 1 if response was 'yes', otherwise 0.

[a] Missing information if no mother, no father.

Characteristics of scale:

Number of items	7
Cronbach's alpha	.72
Range	0–7
Mean	4.2
Standard deviation	.9
High score	Told many people
Low score	Told few people
Missing cases	57

Index